CW01095269

HEARTS OF RESILIENCE

How I Overcame
a Heart Transplant and
a Life of Adversity

PHILLIP HARDWELL

Disclaimer: This book details the author's personal experiences with and opinions about heart disease, diet, mental health etc. The author is not a healthcare provider. You understand that this book is not intended as a substitute for consultation with a licensed healthcare practitioner, such as your physician. Before you begin any healthcare programme, or change your lifestyle in any way, you will consult your physician or another licensed healthcare practitioner to ensure that the examples contained in this book will not harm you.

First printing: 2022

ISBN-13: 9798811217816

British Cataloguing Publication Data:
A catalogue record of this book is available from
The British Library.

To my donor
The hero I've never met

Contents

'Phill is inspirational'

Mark Llewellin, Number 1 best-selling author
who broke the 100-kilometre Treadmill World Record.

Introduction

"The sickest patients that require a transplant are placed on the super urgent waiting list. Phill certainly fulfilled that criteria. Whilst on critical care, he was one of the sickest patients being cared for by the transplant and critical care teams. It's a miracle really and testament to him, his family and the combined efforts of Royal Papworth Hospital teams that we have this outcome."

Richard Quigley, lead nurse for transplants at
Royal Papworth Hospital

I had never believed in miracles. That was until I was lying on a hospital bed in intensive care for 138 days awaiting a life-saving heart transplant and nearly dying three times during that period. As you can tell, the outlook during this period was extremely bleak. There were times when the transplant team could do no more; it was up to my body to fight back and recover well enough to survive an intense number of operations. A miracle was what I needed in order to survive!

My wife at the time was told to prepare to say her goodbyes. However, her response was, "He's not going anywhere." Yes, I was definitely stubborn at times, but no way was I giving up without a fight. Part I of this book takes you through my hospital journey. Somehow, after eight painstaking operations, I made it through this terrifying ordeal and received my new heart. My family were unable to be by my side because of the lockdown caused by the coronavirus pandemic, meaning I had to go through the transplant all on my own.

Amazingly, just two weeks later I was able to walk out of the hospital into the arms of my wife, who was waiting at the entrance, and back to the two boys waiting at home for me to enjoy my second life.

This was not the first time I had been exposed to some form of prolonged suffering. Part II begins in my childhood, where everything looked pretty normal on the outside, while on the inside, alcohol ruled the house. I was a very confused and anxious teenager with no guidance. My mum passed away from heart failure when I was 14; unbeknownst to me until my diagnosis some 15 years later, she had a hereditary type of heart disease with a 50/50 chance of being passed on to immediate family members.

As I grew up, I discovered the sport of bodybuilding when I walked into my local gym and the owner took me under his wing. This resulted in me competing in my first bodybuilding competition at just 15 years of age. Putting my difficult childhood behind me, I joined the military and went on to complete the All Arms Commando Course, one of the toughest military courses in the world, in order to earn the coveted green beret. This was soon followed by exercises in the harsh climate of Norway and over a year serving two separate tours in the war-torn country of Afghanistan.

My resilience came into action again as I was given the news at the age of 29 that I had heart disease. It had seemingly come from nowhere and, just like that, my military career was over. Adjusting to a new career in the civilian world and being severely impacted by my worsening health was extremely tough. As my illness progressed, there were times when I was too ill to walk up the stairs. At that point, a heart transplant was the only option. Combining this with bouts of depression and generalised anxiety disorder throughout my life, it hasn't always been easy for me.

However, the 'never give up' attitude I developed has helped me bounce back time and again to achieve things I never thought possible when I was growing up. I don't think there are any courses out there that teach you how to be more resilient – it is something that is already inside us all. Our mind is the greatest asset we possess. Suffering is not something we should seek to avoid so much as be prepared for, so that when the time comes, we are ready for it and able to react accordingly by not letting it take control of our lives

Throughout my life, my saviours have been regular exercising and eating well. There are endless benefits to both, and without them, I don't think I would be here today.

After the transplant, which I talk about in part III, there were a lot of challenges to deal with, both physically and mentally: spending the best part of a year shielding because of the pandemic; the effect on my mental health; the illnesses I suffered as a result of being immunosuppressed; and the adverse side effects of my medication. No matter how bad life can be, there is always a reason to be hopeful every day. Unexpected events, like my illness, can happen, and it would have been easy for me to play the victim and give up. But I refused. I kept pushing, day by day, and nowadays I view what happened as a reminder for me to develop a deeper gratitude for life and understand what real happiness looks like.

Being able to wake up every day is a blessing and an opportunity to change how we feel about ourselves and improve each day. Now I am extremely grateful and thankful for each waking day, and it's all because of my heart donor and their family for allowing me to continue on with this wonderful life for a while longer.

Although I will never be as fit as I was before the transplant, I reflect on how being so ill that I couldn't walk to then being able to run a half-marathon less than 18 months after my transplant is testament to what the human body and the mind can achieve.

My hope is that when you read this book, my story will inspire you to have a more purposeful life by becoming more resilient, as well as showing you the incredible story of organ donation. By passing on the advice I have learnt through my experiences, through adversity and through bouncing back, my aim is to help others and give something back. As for me, thanks to a complete stranger I have received the greatest gift of all: the gift of life, and a second chance at life, denied to so many. I feel I have a duty to share my story and help others to have a more positive outlook on life.

Part I

Five Months in Papworth: My Biggest Struggle So Far

"He has had eight different trips to theatre during the course of his care before being able to undergo his transplant...He had already waited for a donor organ for several months on an artificial heart support at Royal Papworth and then the COVID-19 crisis hit. We thought we might not get any donors during this time because intensive care units are so stretched in terms of staff and beds. It is a real tribute to the donor's family, and to the hospital from where his donor came, that they had the capacity to think of organ donation while all that we see every day in the news was happening around them."

Mr Pedro Caterino, clinical lead for transplant at Papworth Hospital

It Can Happen to Anyone

First of all, I need to be totally honest with you. Up until the age of 29, the words 'heart disease' had never crossed my mind. I was a fit and active lad serving in the military and in the prime of my life. I had heard stories about it in the media from time to time but I very rarely felt unwell so I thought it was something I may not have to worry about until I was a lot older. How wrong was I!

Excuse my naivety, but I believed heart disease was caused by being overweight, leading a sedentary lifestyle and eating too much saturated fat. I knew from school that eating too much bad fat can clog up the arteries and cause a heart attack. Yes, that may hold true for coronary artery disease, and yes, there is a good reason why we are reminded of this in the news. Coronary heart disease is the most common type of heart and circulatory disease, the most common cause of heart attacks and was the single biggest killer of both men and women worldwide in 2019[1].

Quite a scary prospect, considering there are over seven billion people on the planet.

When the build-up of plaque hardens the arteries, a process known as atherosclerosis narrows or blocks the blood vessels over time and can cause a heart attack or

---

1 British Heart Foundation (July 2021)
https://www.bhf.org.uk/what-we-do/news-from-the-bhf/contact-the-press-office/facts-and-figures

stroke by reducing the blood supply to those areas. The good news is, with the appropriate treatment, a healthy diet, exercise and a good sleep pattern, the progression can be reduced or even prevented altogether.

With that in mind, I had no idea that there are several other heart diseases out there which can be down to a number of different factors.

For example, those you can be born with, known as congenital heart disease, can affect the structure of a baby's heart and how it works. This can range from a small hole in the heart to something more severe; the causes are not always known. There are also inherited heart diseases, which are passed on through families and can begin at almost any age. They could be down to a faulty gene and/or a mutation in one or more of your genes and if one of your parents has this, there is a 50/50 chance it may be passed on to you – which could prove fatal if undetected or left untreated.

Of course, there are several types of heart disease out there and, as I am not a cardiologist, I have just outlined the most common types of heart disease and the inherited type, which is what I had.

While I was serving in the military, I was preparing to compete in a regimental boxing event that happened annually. I enjoyed boxing and keeping fit, so when the opportunity arose that I could take 12 weeks off normal duties to train for this competition – and still be paid – it was a win/win situation!

About four weeks leading up to the tournament, during a routine pad work session, I threw a left hook to my partner. He, rightfully, held his pad up to block it and I felt a snapping sensation in my left bicep. I tried to train around it in the hope that it would heal before the event. Eventually I needed a professional to look at it as it was taking on the appearance of a bruised and deformed plum (only my arm was more swollen!).

After some trips to Southampton General Hospital, I was told I had a ruptured bicep tendon. That meant no boxing competition for me, which I felt gutted about because we had been training two or three times a day and, physically, I was probably in the best shape of my life.

Following what was a fairly routine operation in July 2016 to reattach the bicep tendon to the bone, I woke up confused – and then even more so when I saw a sign above me that read 'Intensive Care Unit'. I hadn't read in the pamphlet that I would end up here, but I told myself it was nothing to worry about.

When I came around properly, woken by the intense pain in my arm from the operation, they told me the news that they had discovered I had an irregular heartbeat. They wanted to keep me overnight and carry out an echocardiogram (ECHO) the next day to check the structure of the heart. So far, nothing to worry about, I thought – so I took up the offer of liquid morphine and got my head down.

The next morning, the cardiology team arrived and carried out an electrocardiogram (ECG) and an ECHO to check my heart for any abnormalities. It turns out I had something called an atrial flutter. This is an abnormal heart rhythm that starts in the atrial chambers of the heart. It can cause the heart to beat too fast or skip beats, which in the past I thought could be attributed to drinking too much coffee or burning the candle at both ends, as they say.

It's not usually life-threatening and can be treated with a procedure called an ablation, which I would become all too familiar with. The procedure involves moving small thin catheters up through the femoral vein in the groin in order to access and effectively be able to destroy the faulty tissue of the heart that is causing the irregular heartbeats.

My time in Larkhill at the Royal School of Artillery was coming to an end and I would soon return to my parent unit, 29 Commando Regiment Royal Artillery in Plymouth. So I had two options: to seek further medical treatment at Derriford Hospital in Plymouth or have the procedure in my home town of Bristol. I chose the Bristol Heart Institute (BHI). However, this meant a 17-week wait just to get an appointment. To be on the safe side, I reduced the intensity of the exercise I was doing and didn't notice any adverse symptoms in the weeks before I was seen.

I eventually had the heart ablation in early 2017. I remember the day of the procedure – Friday 24th March – like it was yesterday. I attended alone, as my then wife Roxy was working at the time and I thought it was just another appointment. But then they called me through to the treatment room, where the lead cardiology nurse and lead cardiologist at the BHI sat me down and broke the news that would change my life forever.

"Phillip, you have Arrhythmogenic Right Ventricular Cardiomyopathy." I had no idea what this was. I was in complete shock and the words said to me during that whole meeting were a blur. Thankfully, they gave me a booklet with great detail about the condition and what I should and shouldn't do. The appointment lasted a couple of hours, and then they let me go home to try and comprehend what I had been told.

Arrhythmogenic Right Ventricular Cardiomyopathy – ARVC – is a rare form of heart disease that is caused by a change or a mutation in the genes. It can be passed on through families but, unlike me, some people can carry this gene with it never developing into full blown ARVC.

This disease causes the proteins that usually hold the muscle cells of the heart together to not repair properly. They eventually become detached and, in an attempt to repair the cells, fatty deposits build up in their place. This stretches the walls of the ventricle, meaning the heart doesn't pump blood around the body as effectively. Over time, this results in a thickening of the right side of the heart and causes abnormal heart rhythms, which were to become quite regular for me.

The tests I'd had done up to now were backed up by my mother's death certificate, which confirmed that she died of Arrhythmogenic Right Ventricular Dysplasia. (Dysplasia and Cardiomyopathy are often used interchangeably for this condition.) Up until this point I had never known the true cause of my mother's death, as I'll explain later on in the book.

This is a condition that isn't treatable and can progressively get worse over time. "Will I still be able to serve in the army?" I asked.

"Probably not," was their response, letting me down gently.

I walked away from that meeting with those four letters ARVC spinning in my head. They would change the course of my aspirations, and life as I knew it.

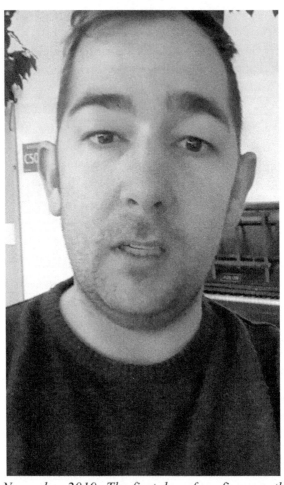

November 2019: The first day of my five-month stay in hospital. I'm carrying approximately 14kg of excess fluid build-up.

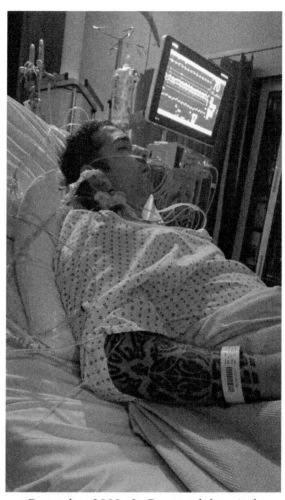

December 2019: In Papworth hospital.
By now things had gone downhill rapidly.

Perilous Times

After that fateful appointment, things remained stable for the next few months. In September 2017 I was fitted with an Implantable Cardioverter Defibrillator (ICD) as a precautionary measure, because living with ARVC increases the risk of Sudden Cardiac Death (SCD). It consists of a small metal box, about the size of a cigarette packet, inserted into the left upper chest area with, in my case initially, a single lead that passes through a vein to the heart, and acts as a pacemaker. This detects any abnormal heart rhythms and relays the recordings through the ICD and a home monitor, which is then sent on to the hospital. This wonderful little box delivers an electric shock if the heart beats too fast or too erratically, a condition known as ventricular tachycardia (VT), which became my arch nemesis. I've heard other people describe the shock as being like a horse kicking you in the chest. Fortunately, I didn't experience this, despite going through several episodes of VT and dizziness, although it must've been close several times. If you are extremely unlucky, the ICD can almost malfunction and go off several times – which sounds really painful!

Thoughts kept running around in my head. How had I gone from running a half-marathon in just over 90 minutes in 2016 to this rapid decline, which, by late 2019, left me struggling to carry out basic tasks and barely able to leave the house? After a great career in the military, having two wonderful boys and meeting Roxy who, at the time, was the woman of my dreams, my recurring low self-esteem and depression had reared its ugly head again. Life was going great until the diagnosis, but you never know when life is going to punch you in the face.

The year 2019 was spent in and out of hospital as I suffered various issues with my heart, which got worse and more serious as time progressed. Ventricular tachycardia is a fast heart rhythm that begins in one of the ventricles of the heart, and it can come as short bursts of a rapidly rising heart rate, as well as longer episodes that can be fatal. I would best describe it as feeling like your heart is beating by your throat and you struggle to breathe, along with feeling dizzy and lightheaded. In the UK, a bout of VT means you must surrender your driving licence for six months minimum, so I had to rely on Roxy to take me to and from work, as well as the numerous hospital appointments that I had to attend. In June of that year I was given the news that I would need a heart transplant, as the damage by then was quite severe, so I went to the Royal Papworth Hospital, world renowned as the leading heart and lung transplant hospital in the UK, to be assessed for suitability. After two days of vigorous tests I was placed on the transplant list.

Roxy and I were getting married at the end of August and, lo and behold, we were in hospital again a week before the big day. Back then, there was no way we were going to miss that date, so the hospital scheduled an operation for a week after the wedding in order for my ICD to be upgraded to a Cardiac Resynchronization Therapy Device (C-RTD). This one helps to treat heart failure and I now had three leads going to my heart, helping it beat more effectively and in sync. This gave me a new lease of life but was sadly short-lived.

It was a wet and dreary November afternoon, a Friday to be exact. The temperature was most likely quite mild for that time of year; however, because I was going through severe heart failure I always felt cold. This was because my body was going into survival mode and keeping the blood mostly around my vital organs, meaning my extremities felt like blocks of ice 24/7.

By this stage of my diagnosis, I was confined to a wheelchair as I felt unable to walk further than 50 metres. When out and about, I struggled by, using a wheelchair and mobility scooter. I became scared, as my independence was fast fading. Since the last time I had seen some of my friends and work colleagues, I had become a shadow of my former self.

Roxy was with me throughout my journey from diagnosis until a few weeks before the heart transplant. Her mind was as sharp as steel and she was immensely strong, both physically and mentally. She was always on hand and ready to recognise any signs that I was regressing further. But she only weighed about seven stone, so how could I expect her to push me around everywhere, as well as looking after our son Luca, who was only 18 months at the time, and working a full-time job? I felt like a burden at times – not myself at all – and my depression was at an all-time low.

My thoughts were, "I should be able to support and provide for my family. Now it is my wife who is looking after me, and I'm only 31."

That Friday was to be my last day of freedom before being confined to a hospital bed for 157 days. It came unknowingly but, at the same time, it was hardly surprising.

On that November afternoon we went to the BHI for a regular appointment. All it took was the panic-stricken face of the cardiologist to suggest that I needed urgent treatment – and fast. My skin looked very grey and clammy, plus I looked like I had gained a severe amount of weight. I hadn't really noticed it myself, as I preferred not to look in the mirror, not only because I was a shell of the man I once was, but also it required a lot of energy for me. We caught a glimpse of my medical history notes; the folder was bursting to the seams at that point.

I was admitted to the Coronary Care Unit. The aim over the next week or so was to hook me up with some diuretic medications via an intravenous (IV) drip and drain the excess fluids that I was holding, and boy, there was a lot! I was normally around 70kg, but for that hospital stay I came weighing in at 84kg! My jeans were now of the skinny variety and my wedding ring was cutting off the circulation to my finger. I reported that I hadn't urinated in the last couple of days and when I did, it came out as a brown trickle. This is a strong indicator of kidney failure, which is a common side effect of severe heart disease. My heart and body were giving up but my mind was staying positive and I thought I would be home in time for Christmas!

Roxy was my guardian angel throughout my journey. She could tell that I was not going to make it to see Christmas without serious intervention, so she phoned the transplant coordinator at the Royal Papworth Hospital several times a day to check when there was a bed available for me.

Thankfully, her persistence finally paid off and, 10 days later, we made the three-plus hour journey to Papworth in the back of an ambulance. For some reason I still kept thinking I would have the transplant and be back home in time for Christmas. Who was I kidding? I was in no fit state to go anywhere.

My Nine Lives

The next six weeks or so were a mixture of fear, delusion and, ironically, a sense of peace. Almost like I had become acquainted with the fact that death was inevitable soon and I may not stay around that much longer. In the back of my mind though, I had this feeling that it was not my time to go yet. I can't recall going down for the eight operations during this short spell of time. I was only informed about what I had been through afterwards, via Roxy and the transplant team. It's probably for the best I didn't know about them at the time, as it would have induced more stress.

Somebody was definitely watching down on me during that period. I vaguely remember early on in December telling Roxy that I felt like I was dying. This was accompanied by bouts of projectile vomiting and I wasn't able to lift my arms at all.

Around this time, I recall setting an alarm to wake me in the early hours so I could watch the Anthony Joshua fight. I didn't make it that far, as one of the doctors came into my room and told us: "We need to carry out an operation tonight or you will probably die." I was really confused and disorientated by now, and most likely unaware of the seriousness of what had just been said to me. I had no other option but to sign the consent form and allow them to take me down to theatre later that night.

That life-saving op involved fitting a machine known as a Biventricular Assist Device (BiVAD), often called an artificial heart. We had a lovely story for my eldest son Reggie that I was like Ironman and I had been given a bionic heart while they were looking for a new heart, frozen in a box somewhere in the hospital! I was fitted with it because by now, both sides of my heart were severely failing.

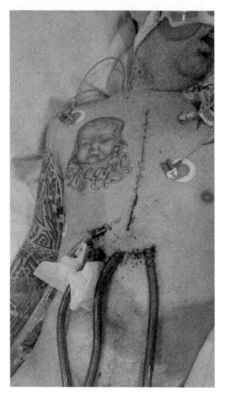

December 2019: How I made it this far is incredible. The four BiVAD tubes are attached to my heart and connected to two machines that circulated blood around my body, as my heart alone was too weak to do so.

The BiVAD consisted of two pumps implanted on each lower ventricle side of my heart, which helped to pump blood from the heart and lungs and around my body, as both sides of my heart were too weak. It is often referred to as a bridge to transplantation. In other words, no going back from here on! The two pumps were connected via four tubes that protruded out of my stomach to two quite hefty machines on a trolley next to me. I had this up until I had my new heart and it is really amazing how these machines work.

I also had another big problem – my lungs were also failing. So I was down to theatre again not too long after to be fitted up to an Extracorporeal Membrane Oxygenation (ECMO) machine. This is a highly specialised piece of equipment similar to the heart-lung bypass machine used for open heart surgery – and only used as a last resort.

From that day on I do not remember anything until a day or so before Christmas. I was heavily sedated from trips to theatre and placed on life support for ten days to let my lungs recover enough on their own to be taken off the ECMO machine.

Now the order of the operations I had no idea about; even if I was with it during these six weeks, it was just too much to take in. All I have been told is that when I returned to the ICU, the oxygenator I had been fitted with to assist with my breathing cracked! This meant I had a lack of oxygen to my vital organs and I went into respiratory arrest. Cardio pulmonary respiration (CPR) via a machine was administered and carried out for around 15 minutes. They later told me they thought I was gone, or I may have suffered brain damage, but thanks to the team I survived to live another day.

On another occasion my left lung began filling up with blood. I can't recall why exactly; at one point I suffered with several blood clots in my central line that had to be suctioned out by one of the nurses. The central line consisted of a catheter placed in one of the large veins to the heart to administer medication and other fluids. It turns out that when I bled, I bled a lot, so a thoracotomy was carried out to access the left lung and drain the blood from it. I still feel numbness on that left side where they had to cut through nerves and muscle.

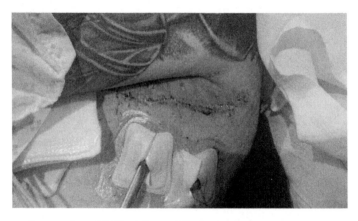

December 2019: After suffering respiratory arrest, the surgeons had to perform a thoracotomy in order to drain the blood from my left lung.

During another operation, I nearly bled to death because my platelets were being destroyed by the BiVAD machine, meaning they wouldn't clot effectively. I was told that I had received over 130 units of blood during that five-month stay, so if you donate blood, I thank you from the bottom of my old and new hearts.

While I was sedated on drugs such as fentanyl and

ketamine, I was completely delusional and my subconscious mind was picking up on many external influences, from the news on the TV to people chatting around me. I became paranoid that everyone was out to kill me, and I had some other frightening delusions that felt so real at the time and were related to events that had genuinely happened in the outside world; however, I was putting my own crazy interpretation on them from all the sedatives.

I have heard stories where people say their life flashes before their eyes when they survive death. I honestly believe that there were two incidents where I was being chased by someone unknown, somewhere in the hospital, and when the chase was eventually up, I succumbed to my mortality. At this point, blood would cover my vision, much as at the beginning of a James Bond movie. However, this was no movie. It felt like life was slowly being sucked out of me and I cannot believe how real it felt.

Throughout my journey to heart transplant, Roxy stayed with me in Bristol until the first Coronavirus pandemic lockdown started on 23rd March 2020. Even then, despite the country being on lockdown, Roxy managed to stay in a local bed and breakfast close to the hospital, waiting in anticipation of any news regarding a transplant. She was great at understanding all the technical knowledge that the doctors and nurses tried to give me, which usually went over my head! She was there to break it down into manageable chunks for me. She brilliantly stuck to the idea of questioning everything that was or wasn't happening. There were times when I was just too tired to argue or confront anybody, so she was like my protector, and was often mistaken for a nurse herself because of everything she picked up during our time there. She definitely left a lasting impact on some of the staff there!

One time, Roxy saved my finger. While in the induced coma, my extremities were freezing throughout and the tip of my right index finger developed necrosis. This may have been because I got frostnip in that finger following a military exercise in the north of Norway, with temperatures of sometimes more than -30 degrees! Since then I have had a painful, tingling sensation in that finger when exposed to cold weather. The nurses didn't seem too concerned with this necrosis developing; their main focus was keeping me alive. Roxy continually pushed the point that, if left untreated, it could lead to infection or even sepsis, which would definitely keep me off the transplant list! I was given antibiotics shortly afterwards to stop any further necrosis.

After my three near death experiences, around the middle of January I was able to sit up again! Albeit only briefly, but it was enough for me to begin using some bike pedals that the physio team brought into my room. This was the start of the comeback and I felt a little bit better and got stronger each day. I still had a feeding tube, which was very uncomfortable, and my weight went from 84kg to 59kg in around two months!

Following the operations to fit the BiVad and ECMO machines, I was considered too unwell to go through a heart transplant operation and had been taken off the transplant waiting list However, towards the end of January we received one of the best pieces of news that I had heard in a very long time. I was to be put back on the transplant list. Not only this, but the super urgent transplant list! This meant that I was the number one priority in the UK to receive a new heart that was a suitable match. It's nice to be first at something for once, I guess!

Things progressed and I managed a short walk each day, and I was able to wash myself daily and shave. Most importantly, the feeding tube came out, but I had to learn how to chew food again. Something we take for granted had to be built up from scratch. I started with soft foods, such as yoghurts and soup. I can't describe the amazing satiety and feeling you get from eating food again after eight weeks without it! Eventually, I got a bit fed up with the hospital food so we used to order a Deliveroo that Roxy would pop down to the foyer to collect. Let's just say, some of the nurses watching me that night were slightly jealous about the aroma of this delicious food!

All was going well until I had a further setback that took me off the transplant list again for two weeks. It started when I woke up in the middle of the night, throwing up relentlessly and with the worst headache known to man. It's one of the most painful things I've had to endure to this day. An MRI scan later confirmed it was a subarachnoid haemorrhage, which could become potentially life threatening. I was given a medication called Nimodipine, which was taken every four hours for ten days to reduce this blood clot in my brain. Gradually, the clot disappeared and my headaches vanished. I was able to go back on the super urgent transplant list once again!

After a few missed opportunities where either a heart had become available but it was an unsuitable match, or I was temporarily off the transplant list, my luck was about to change. A suitable donor had become available.

Now or Never

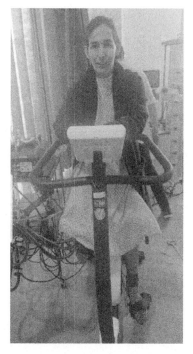

February 2020:
Getting stronger each day

For privacy reasons, very few details are given to patients about the identity of the donor. This is totally understandable, both for the patient, but also to protect the donor's family. Their selfless decision to allow a family member to become an organ donor at a time of huge loss is incredible. A year after my transplant, I wrote to my donor family to thank them so much and let them know they are in my thoughts each day. And that is why, throughout this book, I haven't given any specific dates in case the donor can be identified through death records.

At around 1.30am on an April morning during the midst of the first UK lockdown, one of the transplant nurses came into my room with the news I had been waiting 132 days for. "Phil, the heart we have found for you is a match. So now we are waiting on a coronavirus test that was taken from the donor to come back negative. Once the condition of the heart has been checked thoroughly, the transplant team will retrieve it."

I was overcome with emotion with the news that I was to be given a second chance at life. It was very surreal for me in that room over the next few hours.

People have always dreamed about winning the lottery, along with all the riches they could acquire with it. This was my lottery. Nothing else mattered in life then apart from my health, my family and the friends who had supported us. However, a feeling of guilt overwhelmed me that someone had to pass away in order for me to keep on living, and this plagued my mind for a few months after the transplant.

I had to keep being reassured that if the heart didn't go to me, it would have gone to someone else. This helped somewhat, but to this day I keep asking myself questions such as "What was my donor like?" and "Did I gain any of their personality traits once their heart was inside me?" This phenomenon is known as 'cellular memory', where a transplant patient can sometimes take on the characteristics of the deceased donor. The jury is still out on this one, as everyone is different, and I can't say for sure whether I have lost any of my own or gained any of my donor's personality. Transplant patients have, in the past, developed new personality traits or even taken on food preferences they didn't have before and their donor did. However, this could be because of all the medication, which can alter the taste buds slightly.

The average rate that a heart transplant will be successful during surgery is nine out of ten. I was told about a month or so before I had the operation that my chances of making it through stood at seven out of ten. However, after all that I had been through, that was a risk I was more than willing to take. By that stage I had been far too ill to be considered for transplant on two occasions, a total of eight to ten weeks waiting. If I never recovered well enough again to be suitable for a transplant, there would be no other option available to me but to naturally succumb to this horrible disease.

The protocol was that the transplant patient and the individual who had died had to produce a negative Covid test each to ensure that the organ was still suitable for transplantation and didn't have coronavirus. Now I panicked yet again because we had to wait 24 hours for the result of the first coronavirus test, only for it to come back as inconclusive! I had to wait another agonising 24 hours for another test, which thankfully came back negative. Phew! I felt extremely lucky at this point, as there were rumours going around the UK that they were to stop transplants altogether because of the rapid rise in hospital admissions due to coronavirus.

The report from the retrieval team was that the heart was still in great condition and was getting ready to be transported to Papworth Hospital. Again, the location of the heart is not revealed for privacy reasons; I knew only that it was located within a two-hour radius so that it was not out of the body for too long for it to be unviable. I just felt blessed that a heart had finally been found.

I phoned Roxy, who was staying in a bed and breakfast a few miles away, and we had a brief discussion; I also talked to my older son Reggie's mum, Stacey. Poor old Reg was still half asleep when I saw him via video call. "It won't be long until we will be playing football again, mate," I told him. That was my dream – not going on holiday or some crazy physical challenge, but just the thought of playing football with my boys kept me fighting every day.

My youngest boy Luca was staying with his childminders, Sheila and Gill. They told me that before I went down to theatre, he woke up shouting, "Daddy!" People say he is the spitting image of me; he must also have some telepathic powers to wake up on that night of all nights!

The nurse who had looked after my care for the last three days was Iqbaal, a very kind gentleman of Pakistani origin. We got on well and would often chat about movies; he had told me about the movie *Heat*, starring Robert De Niro and Al Pacino, which was his favourite. "Good choice," I thought; the impression of him pretending to fire a machine gun, maybe not so much! Looking back, I shared some great and surreal times with some of the nurses under my care. They saw me at my worst, cleaned up after I defecated in the bed. The procedure was three nurses would roll me to the side to change the sheets.

Iqbaal would often pray in the room behind me. That night he prayed for me to make it through the procedure safely. He is just one of the many staff, from the surgeons, doctors, nurses to caterers and cleaners, who all play a vital role in making Royal Papworth such a wonderful transplant hospital.

I, too, was praying that night. Although I'm not religious, I do believe that God had been looking over me for the past few months. I have heard a saying along the lines of 'God saves his bravest battles for his strongest soldiers.' I had been through a lot of suffering in my 32 years but I wasn't done giving up yet. I still had plans for the future. My mission was still to be the best father possible for my boys.

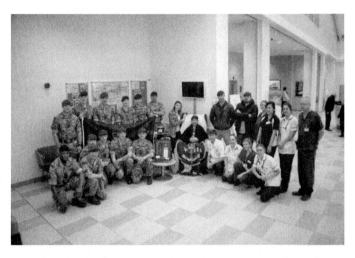

A special day in February when my army friends travelled up to visit, along with the amazing staff at Papworth Hospital

In my hands I held a large framed picture that my 29 Commando regiment friends presented to me when they travelled up to Papworth to visit me back in February that year. It was a great story that made it onto the local television news – plus the sight of up to 13 men in army uniform walking around the hospital turned a few heads, for sure! Sealed in the frame is a black Fairbairn-Sykes Commando dagger, along with The Commando Prayer in full. I recited that prayer dozens of times while waiting to go down for the operation. It got more and more powerful each time I read it.

I had been nervous and apprehensive about this operation, partly because of all the previous complications I'd been through. However, now I was pumped and ready for it. Almost like an elite athlete getting ready before a big competition. I was in the zone and there was not one seed of doubt in my mind that anything would go wrong. I had already visualised myself waking up at the other end of this operation and I had full trust in the team under my care.

As I was wheeled down to the operating theatre, the last thing I remember was the anaesthetist saying that I would slowly drift off. My last thought was about my boys. "I love you, boys. Daddy will be back soon."

Part II

My Journey Pre-Transplant

Growing Up in a
Toxic Environment

Looking in from the outside world, you would sense that I had a fairly normal childhood. I grew up in a three-bed semi-detached house in a small town north of Bristol – a dream location compared to some of the places where I have stayed in the past, both home and abroad.

Until I was 13, I grew up with both my parents. I had a brother called Darren and sister Alison, both older than me, four and six years respectively. There was also another frequent member in our household and it ruled the family. Its name was alcohol.

It came in many forms, from the clear liquid of vodka to the green glass bottles of wine, but its outcome was always the same. It was ever present in our house and it definitely made its presence felt through its consumption by others.

My parents were both heavy drinkers, not so much going to the pub, but more the staying at home and drinking every night type of drinkers. It became apparent to me that it was a big problem when I was about nine. At around the ages of 10-12, the atmosphere in the house became extremely hostile. There would be arguments that increased in intensity as time went on. Whenever I became intrigued or went down to get something to eat, I was shouted at and told to get to my room. I guessed that dinner was off the table at that point.

It was apparent that my mother was drinking and smoking most of the day. Up until the last few years I knew her, she would slur her speech and close herself away in her room most of the time. Maybe that was her safe space? My dad was a functioning alcoholic. He went to work every day and grafted hard. I would have loved to know what the sober version of my mum was like. It was a side that unfortunately I don't have many memories of. I would love to show her the things I have achieved, which I'm sure would make her proud. I'm sure she tried her best in the circumstances she was in, but she couldn't fight the addiction on her own.

My mum worked in various local shops in the town, spending a limited amount of time in each. Often alcohol was the deciding factor that affected this. I remember she was very small and frail in stature but could also stand up for herself when she wanted.

As a young teenager I looked older than my years and I always helped her out when it came to getting her what she wanted. That usually consisted of cigarettes and alcohol. She smoked up to 40 cigarettes a day, possibly more.

My junior school was adjacent to the back garden of our house, and the family dog Jordan would often climb through a hole in our fence and run onto the school playground. Everyone at school thought this was hilarious, and I enjoyed it because it gave me time off a class in order to drop him home again. I'm not quite sure in this day and age you would be allowed to leave school at the age of nine or ten to drop your dog off on your own, but I guess it was a little bit more relaxed back then.

The sight of my dog running around the playground attracted a crowd and I loved being the centre of attention. It was a far cry from the shy awkward teenager I grew to become. Come to think of it, maybe I was always trying to seek approval from others as I wasn't getting this at home? I remember acting the fool at times just to get others to like me, which embarrasses me now. Looking back, I relied on the validation of others in order to feel good. In reality, I wasn't being true to my real values, which were to study hard and exercise.

I recall on one of these occasions when I dropped my dog off at home, I found my mum sitting in her usual armchair in the living room, unable to move. I knew she had some mobility issues from time to time but this time it was apparent that she was clearly drunk, and it had not gone past 11am. On the side of the fireplace was a packet of cigarettes, which I believe my dad put there, knowing she would be unable to get off her chair and reach them. When she saw me, she asked me to pass her the cigarettes, almost begging in a way to suggest that she needed one along with the alcohol to satisfy the demons. Intrigued, I grabbed one out of the packet, put it in my mouth and tried lighting it, but to no avail. I didn't realise at that age that you had to breathe in for it to light properly. I remember the awful taste of the burning cigarette, so I quickly passed the packet to my mum, we made a pact and I went to school without telling anyone about it… Until now. They say you are a product of your environment and it would be only a matter of time before I was smoking and drinking for real.

I always felt a sense of jealousy of the other kids at school, even my closest friends. We would go to the park and play football after school for as long as the daylight hours let us. Afterwards, it was back to our homes – theirs all well-kept with a loving and supportive family, while mine, on the other hand, was not a safe, warm and loving place.

I'd come back to the sight of my mum passed out drunk at the bottom of the stairs. I had no idea what had happened beforehand. All I knew was that this must have been the result of another all-day drinking session. She would often wet herself, totally unaware of what had gone on. My brother and sister were often out with their friends and it was usually up to me and my caring nature to carry her upstairs to bed.

My dad didn't really care too much at this time. He was out working all day, only to come home to find my mum in a drunken state by teatime. I imagine that many of the arguments started this way and my dad wasn't usually good at expressing himself, thus ensuring many angry blazing rows. My sister had pretty much moved out by this point, which I can't blame her for. But I didn't really have a choice in this situation. As you can imagine, hearing your parents fighting makes you want to shut yourself off from the rest of the world and not tell others, as, ironically, I felt to blame for much of it. Was I to blame for my parents' heavy drinking? Definitely not, but it's amazing what the mind can believe if you tell it so.

Fear of Abandonment

I can recall one time when my parents were in the living room during yet another argument. My dad called me down and said, "Phil, go to your mother's room and look for any empty vodka bottles. I will give you £1 for every empty bottle you find." As I walked upstairs, I caught my mum's drunken stare; I could see the terror in her eyes. I'm still able to picture it now even though it was over twenty years ago.

I found a 70ml bottle of vodka hidden in a wardrobe underneath a pile of clothes. My irrational mind got to thinking of all of the possibilities that I could spend that pound on. Sweets or football stickers… but then it hit me. I had this overriding sense of guilt. I didn't want to fuel the fire by bringing this bottle down and I didn't want to see my mum get hurt physically. I did what I thought was morally right. I went downstairs and said: "No, I didn't see any." Often when an argument was on the horizon, it meant it was time to go upstairs and not be seen or heard until the next day, when it would be like nothing had happened.

My dad seemed to handle his drinking slightly better, or at least have some limitations. His job as a carpenter kept him busy during the day and enabled him to escape from the chaos at home. He used to smoke but managed to give up before the blazing arguments became more frequent. I think he held it against my mum that she still smoked heavily, as well as drinking too much and having all day in order to do it. Instead of them trying to seek help from one another or externally, there was only resentment and anger towards each other.

There wasn't a lot of love and support to be found in our household. A lack of communication meant there was no "How are you feeling?" or "How was your day?" It was almost like we all went our separate ways and lived different lives. This meant that, as children, we weren't really held accountable for anything. There was a distinct lack of discipline in most areas of the house, like whether we cleaned up or if the house was tidy, or even in school if we got in trouble. Back then, I believed that by behaving badly I would get more attention than for doing well. There were no aspirations for us to be successful or have any dreams. I don't think anyone in my family really cared. It's sad, looking back, not to have had that support and guidance through the journey of life.

This lack of guidance meant there was definitely a high risk of me going off the rails and misbehaving. I was no angel growing up but I still knew the difference between right and wrong. I had every excuse in the world to blame my bad behaviour on my upbringing, but it went against my nature a lot of the time. The times I did mess up were mainly with the aim of attracting attention, fitting in, or impressing other people.

I was a product of my upbringing and for that reason I would go around with a chip on my shoulder against anyone who looked like they had it better than me. "Why is everyone else's life better than mine?" I'd think. I had a vendetta against those people who seemed to have a good family life, with all the love and support they could need. In reality, I was jealous and resentful of all these things because I wanted them for myself. However, when it came to getting them, I turned them away because I didn't deem myself worthy enough. I had a classic victim mentality mindset: life was happening to me, not for me. I reacted with this poor attitude and was stuck in a negative feedback loop of going nowhere, repeating the same mistakes and just existing in life.

At about the age of 12, I started smoking and drinking with the mindset that I didn't care. No one else cared about me, so why should I? This later turned to drug taking, starting with weed, then moving on to ecstasy and cocaine. If you share a bedroom with an older brother and five or more of his friends come over regularly and take drugs, then it is only a matter of time before you take them yourself. My brother and his friends, credit to them, tried to hold me off as long as possible, but I was too curious and looked up to them. These illegal substances were far too easy to get hold of, and slowly became rife around the local places we would hang out. At around the age of 13 I eventually got my own room, when my sister moved out, and I carried out the same activities as my brother, but with my friends and some of the older lads I'd met. It's not something I am proud of but it made me feel accepted and part of a group.

Using drugs and alcohol gave me a release from how awful I thought my life was. I'm sure everyone would agree that going around with these kind of destructive thoughts in your head throughout your teenage years while on mind-altering drugs is not a positive start in life for anyone.

A point I want to make is that it's never too late to make a change. Maybe that's why I talk to myself a lot better nowadays and prefer to focus on the positives instead of negatives. This can be more difficult than it sounds. The human brain is more attuned to negative thoughts because it is usually focused on survival mode. We can get stuck in the fight or flight system response. This builds as stress in the body and can affect how we live our daily lives. Over time, we need to change our negative thoughts and beliefs about how we view life and there are little things we can do each day to change it.

The truth of the matter is that every person on the planet has some sort of problem, from the homeless person wondering where the next meal will come from, to the billionaire who can't decide what car to buy next. If the brain doesn't have a problem, it will search for ways to find one. Maybe that's why people argue and put others down on social media; it makes them feel somewhat more entitled than others. Or is it that their brain is bored, so insulting someone fills the void? The point I'm trying to make here is about accepting the fact that we will always have some sort of problem and we need to accept this and not let it take over our lives. Some problems can be out of our control, whereas others can be a direct result of our own actions. Do you think it's better to feel sorry for yourself and further drive yourself into a negative state, worrying about it, or to get up every morning with a fresh start? Stop letting one setback define you as a person. Instead, assess the situation, and learn and grow from it by forgetting about it and taking action every day.

A classic analogy of this is having one flat tyre so you slash the other three. Or 'dieting' in order to lose weight. We tend to go all or nothing, and if we stray from our plan, we tell ourselves we've already failed so we might as well gorge on not-so-healthy foods. We can always start again on Monday – only to trip up again, usually after a bad day or on the weekends.

Nowadays, life has never been more comfortable and plentiful, yet we are more miserable than ever. It doesn't make sense!

I think social media has a lot to answer for. I am so glad that it was not around when I was a teenager. I was constantly comparing myself to others and what they had and if there had been social media, I feel it would have exacerbated things even more.

The problem with social media is not only that it is super addictive, but it is only looking at a snapshot of someone's life. For example, that influencer with the perfect body and lots of money? They still have problems. Some may be suffering with mental health issues themselves. We often compare ourselves to the impossible and feel disappointed when we can't achieve these levels. Think of a celebrity you admire, one who is always airbrushed in a photograph. Essentially it is not real life but a modified version of them, but we are tricked into thinking that if we buy this product they are promoting, then we too can look as good as them. Chances are, if you saw them walking down the street, they would probably look a lot different to how they are portrayed in their online photoshoot.

The internet has changed the way we communicate – and not necessarily in a positive way. Nowadays, from the comfort of our own homes we can send messages of abuse to complete strangers in order to try and make ourselves feel better. But instead, ask yourself questions like, "What is the root cause of this anger. Where is it coming from?" You'll usually find it's hidden in your own life somewhere.

We only have one life and one body, therefore we need to embrace our imperfections and accept ourselves for who we truly are. Fall in love with yourself first before loving someone else. I am short and I talked too slowly growing up. People would tease me about this. The slow talking made me think that people thought I was stupid. You think there is something wrong with you, and that life's not fair. It can be hard to process these imperfections as a kid. However, as I grew older, I started to further investigate these unfounded beliefs. I had always focused on the negatives of these 'imperfections', so I began to question these beliefs and slowly accepted myself as I am. So yes, there's nothing I can do about being short; it just means I can spend less money on clothes. Does talking slowly mean that people may undermine my intelligence? I question that thought and remind myself that I have a degree, so I can't be that stupid.

Own it – and remember that no one can talk to you as badly as you have spoken to yourself in the past. Once you ignore the opinions of other people, you will feel a sense of enlightenment. But you wouldn't speak to a friend the way you speak to yourself. This needs to stop; you need to shut up that inner critic, which tells you that you can't be this or that. Start being kinder to yourself. Be grateful for what you do have, because it will be the envy of another person.

Over a long period of time, I gradually began self-acceptance and to embrace the one body I was given. This is one of the keys to developing your own self-confidence, which can make you start feeling a lot better about yourself. Stop searching for external factors, such as material possessions, otherwise you will always be searching for that elusive happiness.

Was It Alcohol
or Something Else?

When I was 14, my mum, who, at the time, had been staying alone at my grandad's house, about 400 metres away from the family home, was found dead, all alone in her bed. The bed she was found in was downstairs, in the living room. By this point she had struggled to move around and was restricted to the downstairs only. When her body was discovered, she weighed about five stone and probably hadn't eaten in weeks. Looking back, I can't imagine the pain and suffering she must have been going through. To this day, I still have a sense of guilt knowing that I would have been the last person to see her alive.

By now I was the only person who popped around to see her and tried to help her. No one else bothered. As you can imagine, there was not much help that I could provide for her. The only help she wanted was in the form of alcohol or cigarettes. I wish I had been mature enough to have phoned an ambulance to get my mum the help she so clearly needed, before it was too late.

The consensus in our household was that our mum was the bad person because she would get blind drunk all the time and not know what she was doing. I felt that we had been somewhat brainwashed by my dad and others into thinking this. He was the breadwinner; he put the food on the table. I think he deeply resented the fact that my mum was not the woman he married, the woman she was before the alcohol took hold. I remember seeing her dead body before the funeral. She was extremely cold to the touch. My first thought was that she was at peace now.

The funeral was a truly emotionless occasion. I wanted to express my emotions, but I didn't know how. Sounds strange, I know, but when you have been keeping your thoughts to yourself your whole life, it can be difficult to open up to others. After the funeral there was a wake at a local pub. I had a few pints of lager and was being my usual quiet and reserved self. I remember getting a lift home afterwards and going up to my bedroom. The combination of other people's pity and the booze sent me into a fit of rage, and I started smashing up my bedroom door. No one else was home yet, but I don't think they would have done anything had they known what I was doing. It felt like a release of all the pent-up emotions I had bottled up that day and for years before.

After my mum's death, life was very awkward for a while. Over the next couple of years, my dad's drinking began to get worse. He would be up late, playing loud music – mostly Whitney Houston – and even loudly singing along. If I ever asked him to turn it down because I had football Sunday morning, I would face a barrage of abuse. It made me want to grow up quicker and get out of there. He was grieving, and I guess drinking and listening to loud music helped his grieving process.

Thankfully, my dad met a new partner and it was good to see him happy again. Life got a bit more stable then, a bit more family-like. Meals at the table, that sort of thing. A little too late though, I thought. However, it was short-lived as Dad and his new partner decided to move to where she lived, about 50 miles away, somewhere in Wiltshire. It would be a fresh start for my dad. He set up an agreement that he would rent the house out to my brother, and Darren would care for me while he was gone – only to return on a Sunday to collect his rent money and leave again.

At the start, this new-found independence felt great. The notion that my brother and I could have a house party on any day and there would be no repercussions felt like a dream come true. How wrong was I!

I was still a child, only 16 years old, and I still needed parental care. My brother was working as a carpenter and supported me at that stage as I was still at school. I started working some evening shifts at a gym called Peak Physique and barely managed to scrape together enough money to pay a small amount of rent and buy food from myself.

I remember when I was growing up, people would ask me about my mum and I was too embarrassed to say that she had died, not only because I was such an awkward kid, but because it made me feel inferior to them, and it was also a sure conversation killer. I had this perception that her dying meant there was something wrong with me.

I would say that I definitely went through some phases of anxiety and depression during my younger life. That fight or flight mode was certainly present when listening to arguments or hearing loud noises downstairs. As an adult, I am more aware of what it is and the symptoms, plus I have spoken out about it and asked for help. In my eyes, that was the start of the healing. I tried healing myself by reading books and writing unrealistic things that I could change about myself but it normally led to me going through cycles of depression. Sometimes I would feel great, confident and full of energy but after a couple of weeks or so, the motivation would subside and I would feel almost unable to muster up the energy to do anything. I would have a couple of days of locking myself away, trying to avoid contact with others and self-loathing in the comfort of my own home. I still have the odd day or so of this, and some days, if I am tired, there's absolutely nothing wrong with taking a day out to relax and catch up on sleep. Burnout can be just as bad as not doing much, so it is important to schedule in some rest days.

If, like me, you get these feelings of depression and hopelessness, try to identify what you are feeling and what you can do to get you out of this situation. A notebook and pen can be your best friend in lifting your mood, along with getting some fresh air.

Back then, mental health was not something that was really talked about, or if it was, you were labelled as different, or even weak. If I had been told I suffered with depression as a kid, I probably wouldn't have believed it. I thought I was just born this way and that I didn't deserve to be happy or as worthy as others. How was I meant to know what mental health was when I had no one to speak to about it growing up? I am glad now that in this day and age, there is more information and support out there so you don't have to feel like you are alone.

If you feel like you are suffering with your mental health, which undoubtedly most of us will at some stage in our lives, don't suffer alone. Reach out to others before it is too late.

Thankfully, I found something that took my mind off things – and I truly believe it helped save my life.

Finding Fitness

Despite the bad hand I was dealt during my early life, there was one positive thing I did find, and I still use it to this day and will do for as long as it's physically possible. Like I said previously, I believe it is the main reason why I am still alive now.

Exercise has been, and still is, very much part of my everyday life.

It can be something small, like going for a walk each day, even if it is raining outside! Yes, I am reluctant at first, but then I think back to the times when I couldn't walk, and that pushes me to go out there and make the most of being able to move again. Plus, with our dog Pedro (named after the surgeon who saved my life!) looking out of the window waiting to go out, I know it will do us both good!

I think there's a common agreement that going out for a walk, especially in nature, makes you feel better than not going out at all. My usual routine during my recovery throughout the lockdowns (when clinically extremely vulnerable patients were advised to stay in as much as possible) involved going out to walk the dog in the morning at about 6am when no one else was about. Then I would move on to the gym I created in the garage. I had built up a good collection of weights and had a nice little set up going on, consisting of free weights, a punch bag and a rowing machine. This meant I literally had to walk about ten metres to get to the equipment I needed to get a decent workout in.

All this was so I could return to something that I had loved and missed so dearly. I had to wait about 12 weeks for my sternum to heal, but that was a small wait compared to the years of exercise I had missed from being so unwell.

During the thoracotomy surgery all the nerves and muscles had been cut through on my left side. This led to me being overly protective of that side and now I had to pay for that by building it back up again to be as good as it is going to get with all the scarring.

I must stress that I started from scratch in getting back to working out. I started out walking just a couple of hundred metres and lifting 1kg weights. It was slow and frustrating but necessary to get my strength and fitness back gradually. The last place I wanted to end up was the hospital!

Life and excuses can always get in the way of keeping fit and healthy. Usually it boils down to a perceived lack of time, which in turn leads to a lack of effective planning of your time. We have more ways in which to exercise, from gyms to sports clubs and our living rooms; however, in this fast-paced life, we have more excuses or distractions than ever at our disposal. Working longer hours, getting distracted watching a TV series, scrolling through social media...

Exercising needs to be made a priority and something that you can enjoy, so we can all make some form of regular exercise part of our daily habits. Even if it's only a walk, done consistently it will bring several great physical and mental health benefits.

Always remember that rest is very important as well. There are times where I have to remind myself that I am not as fit, or ever will be, as I was when I was in the military, so sometimes I need a day or two to fully rest and recharge.

Otherwise I will burn out, which will, in turn, make me unwell for a few days or more.

A lot of my friends play golf, which again is a good form of exercise because of all the walking involved. However, for me, golf is a bit too sedentary as I have always been quite a fidgety person! It's all about finding something you enjoy and doing it consistently. I enjoy running: it helps to clear my head and I feel fantastic afterwards. If you hate running, then it is not something that you are going to stick to long term, especially on a cold wet winter morning!

I first played football for a local club at the age of seven, and I continued until I was 21. This was when the demands of being away a lot with the military meant I couldn't commit to it fully. There were times when I didn't enjoy playing football and I wanted to quit. However, I kept on pushing through, playing and enjoying the training sessions. Before football matches, I would be struck with this overriding fear that I would make a mistake that would lead to me embarrassing myself or the team losing. This would usually subside after about ten minutes, once the game and my own mind had settled down. Looking back, I wish I could have told my younger self that it doesn't matter if you make a mistake. Just go out and have fun! Even if you do make a mistake or lose, no one will remember and it won't matter in time gone by. Failure is simply a lesson to help us learn from our mistakes. However, we all see failure as a bad thing and let it define us.

By chance, I found a new sport that has become a passion for me and helped me to set goals for myself.

Peak Physique

As a kid, like millions of other kids I had a dream of being a professional footballer. I think all my friends did. However, I think I knew it wasn't going to happen. Some would think that is quite negative, but deep down, I knew I didn't have the discipline to reach the level of commitment required. Like I said before, I had a lot of personal issues to deal with after my mum passed away. The impact of her death made me close myself off from the world around me. It was very difficult as a teenager to talk about her death as it made me feel more awkward and I found it easier to say nothing. This, along with discovering alcohol, was my coping mechanism to overcome my low self-worth and block out negative thoughts.

I did have another ambition, and this one wasn't so well-known. It was something I thought I had more chance of success in, or so I thought at the time. Bodybuilding.

From the age of 13, a couple of friends and I would check out a local gym after school. The gym was situated in a row of four or five derelict buildings, which were either empty or used for storage or making materials such as blinds or windows. The row was topped off with a worn-down pub on the corner and flats above each building. The car park was very neglected and not somewhere you would want to leave your car overnight or hang about after hours.

The gym was called Peak Physique. I know there are many others called this all over the world, but this one was definitely unique in its own little way. It was best summed up as your typical spit and sawdust gym, perfect for heavy lifters, where people made grunting noises as weights were chucked around without a care. It was a little less welcoming for females and kids, like we were at the time. Maybe that was what attracted me to the place – it was somewhere I could grow and finally belong. It was great for a young, hungry lad like me who wanted to find some direction in life while grasping the basics of weight lifting.

The gym had a small entrance area where people would congregate to drink protein shakes and chat about work or whether they were going to the local high street that night. (It was full of lovely pubs where everyone knew everyone and you would usually see a fight by the end of the night!) They also sold things like Lucozade and flapjacks, which were loaded with sugar, but because they were being sold in a gym they must have been healthy, right?!

To the right of the gym foyer was the main weights room. This was filled with free weights and cable machines. I don't think it was very welcoming to women, though. Luckily, nowadays we have lots of modern franchise gyms that are more user friendly and inviting to everyone, equipped with high tech machines and offering 24-hour access and classes.

Back into the reception, there was a staircase that led to some cardio equipment, a toilet and some makeshift changing rooms – if you could call them that; I don't think they would be considered suitable for use today! The cardio equipment upstairs consisted of some treadmills, exercise bikes and cross trainers. When they were not out of order, that is. But it was a place of solace for those intimidated by the sound of iron crushing down on the concrete floor below and fully-grown burly men shouting after a heavy set of deadlifts.

The three of us would embark on the mile-long walk to the gym after school, still in uniform and with gym kits in our bags. All young and naive, and without a clue about what we were doing! I wasn't fearful about looking stupid, though, as I was so young compared to the other members and I struck up a good relationship with the gym owner.

At first it was more like a social after school club, and we went out of curiosity and mostly for a laugh. But we persisted and, over time, we got used to lifting weights and carrying out the basic exercises – more than likely with terrible form!

Even though I don't think we achieved much in the first six months of going to the gym, exercising in that kind of intimidating environment was a great introduction to the world of strength training. When it came to lifting weights and being consistent, people would come up to me and say, "You shouldn't be squatting that type of weight at your age. Your spine hasn't fully developed yet." Yes, it may stunt your growth, but when you're dedicated to something and you see continual progression, along with the feeling that it gives you, you tend to forget any of the long-term consequences – if it was true, that is.

Once the messing about stopped, the next period of training proved invaluable in getting to know the basics of how to carry out exercise with good form, what equipment to use, how to train each muscle group and what foods to eat to recover and get stronger. Learning this means that whenever I walk into a new gym, with new faces, I don't feel intimidated, no matter how old or out of shape I am. This is not to sound arrogant because I am quite humble!

But I have built up a solid foundation over many years, so I know what works for me and what doesn't. I usually head to the gym, get my workout in and I'm out in under an hour. My stretching and mobility can be done at home with the dog or Luca climbing all over me!

There were a lot of weird and wonderful characters at the gym, the owner in particular. Rob was what you could call a larger than life character. Inside his gym he was knowledgeable and slightly arrogant, and he had a good physique for a man of his age. Outside the gym he was quite reserved and, in his own words, enjoyed going out 'people watching' around the local area. I recall one time I dropped him in it when I told another gym member that Rob had seen him buy junk food at the supermarket. This guy was not happy in the slightest and pinned Rob against the wall and said, "Are you f***ing watching me shopping?!"

Rob saw potential in me and my friend Baz, and we progressed well. We started training regularly three to four times a week, taking protein and creatine supplements and seeing some good muscle size in the process. I guess you could also call us regulars by now! Rob treated us with a bit more respect, and when we said that we couldn't afford the membership fees of £15 each month, being only 14 years old, he offered us both jobs there. This covered our membership fees and allowed us to train for free whenever we wanted.

In some ways, Rob became a father figure to me. He always offered me extra work so I could get my training sessions in and get away from the depression I faced at home. It meant I could earn a little bit of much-needed income too. Unfortunately, he was too kind in nature and people treated him and the gym disrespectfully. There was no care for the equipment and people would often try to go without paying for membership.

It all came to a head one day when the usual gym goers arrived to carry out a training session, only to find out that the gym had closed! Rob had had enough of operating at a loss and people taking advantage of him, so he decided to close up and get away from it all. I couldn't blame him really; he was getting close to retirement and I guess the toll of it all wasn't worth the stress.

I felt gutted that Peak Physique had closed. It was the gym that I had become accustomed to, a gym that sometimes had no heating, where people in baggy clothes would go to lift heavy weights.

After about ten years of training, it felt like the end of an era. It was time to find a new gym and keep the momentum going. But long before the closure, all the enjoyment I gained from weight training had improved my self-esteem and made me want to challenge myself further. So much so that my next goal was to enter a bodybuilding competition at only fifteen years of age!

Mr Wales?!

As I got more and more into weight training and working out at the gym, I heard the news that there were people in the gym who competed in natural bodybuilding competitions. I read about the professional bodybuilding competitions in magazines such as *Flex* and *Muscle & Fitness*, which were scattered around the gym. I was amazed by the size and strength of some of these professional bodybuilders and I wanted to be like them, almost – I didn't know what they were taking to get to that size and had no idea what steroids were, back then. Word had got around that I was this kid with good size and shape for his age who knew what he was doing. So I thought to myself, "Why don't I try it myself? What have I got to lose?"

I set myself a challenge. I signed up to compete in the Mr Wales under 18s category amateur bodybuilding competition. I would have been 15 at the time of entering but I felt ready for the under 18s category despite only having around two years' training under my belt. This gave me focus and allowed me to train that little bit harder, knowing that I would be on stage wearing just a thong and posing in front of hundreds of people! People say that public speaking is their number one fear, but being on a bodybuilding stage can be scarier. And no, it is not baby oil; it is usually the sweat reflecting off the beams of the lights shining down on you!

I would wake up about 6:30 in the mornings and complete some cardio on an empty stomach. This consisted of either running or cycling. Eating on a budget meant lots of eggs, tuna, bread, milk and pasta, as well as protein shakes, which were taken in abundance. I'd have four boiled eggs and oatmeal for breakfast and make a tuna and sweetcorn sandwich with wholemeal bread for my school lunch, along with an apple. Dinner would consist of a chicken breast and pasta with some spices, as well as a protein shake after training. That was pretty much my routine for the 12 weeks leading up to the competition. Pretty hardcore for a 15-year-old, but I was committed to proving a point to myself and those who had doubted me up until this point in my life. I don't recall anyone in my family asking how I got on. They were unaware of the time and effort it took for me to prepare for the competition, so it did hurt when they didn't want to watch or even ask about it or encourage me.

I had always put on muscle easily but I found losing fat difficult. I would read bodybuilding magazines in the gym and notice these amazing-looking products that included a secret ingredient to get ripped. They were marketed excellently and I was taken in by the fact that these fat burners were available. The pictures would always show very ripped athletes promoting the products. I was drawn into them like a fly to a lightbulb. With all these fancy words such as 'catalyst' and 'annihilate fat', I was convinced that this was the missing ingredient I needed to get that all-aspiring six-pack. Bottom line, like anything worthwhile in life, there are no quick fixes and results take time!

Looking back now, it's crazy that my whole life was defined by believing that I needed a six-pack in order to be accepted and successful. I always thought that by having one, it would open up the gateway to other opportunities in life… mainly attraction from the ladies and all the trappings that being in shape brought with it, or so I thought. I was basing my values on extrinsic values and seeking approval from others. I wasn't thinking intrinsically and doing it because I wanted to, which is probably why I didn't have a six-pack for long – plus I loved food!

This, however, called me to obsess over eating and I would go through periods where I would severely restrict my calorie intake in order to lose as much fat as possible. What I know now is that this is not sustainable long-term. At the weekends or after a couple of weeks of restrictive eating, I would fall off the waggon and eat every sweet and fatty treat in sight. To counteract this, I would do extra cardio in the gym and take these so-called fat burners, thinking they would get me back into a low body fat percentage. A lot of the fat burners on the market today are really just pumped with caffeine, which gives you a lot of energy to work out and increases your heart rate. I suppose it makes you feel like you can push harder and burn more fat. If that's the case then why not have a black coffee before a workout for a fraction of the price!

This constant cycle of yo-yo dieting, as it's more commonly known, stayed with me for a lot of my adult life. It wasn't until I found out more about it that I realised it was emotional eating – because that's exactly what I was doing. I had this perfectionist mindset that meant if I had one bad treat then the whole diet would be ruined and I would start all over again, only to repeat the cycle. Often when I was having these binges, I wasn't really taking the time to enjoy the food or process it; it was almost like it was my subconscious mind and bad habits that would make me eat out of sadness or boredom. It's not until you become more conscious of what you are eating and become more mindful that you can change your approach to losing weight.

At the time it felt like a sense of comfort from something else I was lacking in life. Maybe it was a lack of love and support growing up. All I knew was that food was always there for me and it would shift my moods. That is, until after the binge when I felt like crap.

If this sounds familiar and something you may be doing, then I wouldn't be afraid to seek help to understand the underlying reasons why you are overeating. My top advice is to change your approach and have a strategy when it comes to food. You can have the best diet in the world but if you don't address the root causes for why you overeat – the triggers or obstacles you face – you will not stick to it in the long term. First of all, don't restrict any foods. That means if you want a kebab then have one – and enjoy it! Someone who is in control of their eating habits will know that no foods are off limits and will enjoy eating foods knowing they can balance the calorie intake over the course of a week. You will have some good days where motivation is high and you feel inspired, and bad days where you are tired and unhappy. On these days, the brain will seek out these pleasure foods and quick fixes to make you feel better. That's why I don't keep certain foods in the house. Chocolate is a prime example!

On 4th August 2002, aged 15, we set off to Porthcawl in South Wales for the Mr Wales bodybuilding competition. This was also a qualifying event for the Mr Great Britain competition, to be held later that year. Ironically, I didn't feel nervous whilst I was on stage, despite my usual shy and reserved nature. Maybe this was because I had put in the effort to look good, and I prepared, mentally, as best as I could, knowing what I knew at the time with the tools that I had. If you know deep inside that you have done all you can to prepare, that gives you a certain inner confidence with which to succeed.

I also felt I had prepared as best as I could for the training and losing fat side of things. However, when it came to completing the eight mandatory poses and making up a freestyle routine with a combination of poses to a song of your choice for up to two minutes in front of three judges, I was not so good! And that's probably what cost me the Mr Wales title.

There was also a sense of fear, because there were only two in my class and I had watched a video of the competition the previous year. The guy I was up against had competed before, so I assumed he would win because he was more experienced than I was. In a way, I had already accepted defeat. But if I had been more confident and worked more on my posing routine, I think I would have won it. It became a bit of a talking point for me in the future, especially when people assumed that I was Mr Wales! I didn't correct those who said it, which I should have now, looking back. So, if you're reading this thinking I once held the Mr Wales title, please accept my apologies. I never said I won it; I only shyly agreed when someone brought it up!

Regardless of the result, it was a great experience for me at such a young age, and something most of the other gym members hadn't achieved. It was something I thought would never be possible. I was under the illusion that it was going to act as a stepping stone into my future bodybuilding career. Unfortunately, I had a lot of my own demons holding me back that I had to try and juggle too.

The Mr Great Britain competition, which was held in October of that year, consisted of the top two UK qualifiers in each category from each of the five national bodybuilding competitions across the British Isles. As there were only two of us in our category for Mr Wales, it meant I had a place, and a shot at winning Mr Great Britain! The best from the south, the east, the north, Wales and Scotland battled it out for this prestigious trophy. I wanted to enter the competition, but I didn't want to stick with the restrictive diet I had put myself through last time, or the work required to get in shape for it. Besides, I was enjoying my football too much at the time, as well as drinking alcohol on a regular basis.

Despite finding it hard to let people down, I eventually plucked up the courage to tell Rob that I didn't want to compete in Mr Great Britain. He understood and nothing further was mentioned of it. That was up until after the event, when he nonchalantly informed me, "Nobody turned up for the under 18s category so you would have won if you had just shown up!"

What if…? What if I had turned up and ended up being the winner of the under 18s Mr Great Britain bodybuilding competition? Each winner won an all-expenses-paid holiday to Italy to compete in the European Championships! What an amazing experience that would have been – plus I had already written to several bodybuilding supplement companies asking for sponsorship. That would have been an amazing opportunity and could have led to a great career in bodybuilding.

At that age though, my friends and I were going out

drinking and taking drugs regularly, and I didn't have the discipline to choose the bodybuilder lifestyle. In reality, my life was a mess and I was a quitter. If things got tough, I gave up. Nobody told me what to do and I had no one to turn to for advice. I needed something to push me in order to release my inner potential. The new career I was about to embark on would give me that kick up the backside and the shock to the system that I so desperately needed.

A Decision That Turned My Life Around

Up to now, my life had been full of ups and downs. Mostly downs, wallowing in a pit of my own self-pity, and making some bad decisions that had cost me dearly. After I left school, I started and gave up a bricklaying apprenticeship in the first year. I was labouring three days a week and going to college on the other two days of the working week. Back then, it was pretty much the gold standard advice given to most youngsters in my peer group. "Get a trade and you'll be sorted for life," they kept saying. My dad and my brother were both carpenters, but I was pretty useless when working with my hands in an intricate way. In reality, the real reason I gave up was because I was lazy when it came to learning new things and turning up on a consistent basis. I quite enjoyed the manual labour side of building because of the physical aspect involved; the learning side, not so much. I now realise that we shouldn't stop learning as soon as we leave school. If we are continually learning throughout our lives, we are growing as a person, which in turn gives us more purpose in life, which I feel is one of the factors for living a happier life.

After a year of the two-year apprenticeship I didn't bother showing up and I dropped out of the bricklaying course. I had no one to keep me accountable. I needed someone to give me a kick up the backside! Carpentry is a great career but I just didn't feel that it was right for me. I wanted – and really needed – to escape from my hometown and the clutches that drinking and drug-taking had on me, in order to develop myself and explore more of the world.

When I was younger, I had requested a British Army joining pack, the one you could get in the post with all the information about the joining process. Fear of failure had held me back from a lot of things but, at 17, I finally took the plunge and walked into the army career office in the centre of Bristol to register my interest. I had no family members who had served in the military, and to be honest I didn't know a great deal about it either. My mind was set on joining the army, but not on which regiment I wanted to be posted to. They asked me what I was interested in and I whittled it down to three choices: driving, building stuff and big guns. This meant there was the choice of joining the Royal Logistic Corps, the Royal Engineers or the Royal Artillery. The first two had a long waiting list and the Artillery appealed to me the most, not only because of the big guns they used but also because they had commando and parachute regiments, in which I could further test myself. My signing of the oath of allegiance took place in May 2006 and it was the best decision I have ever made.

The lure of being posted to a different country was extremely appealing. I had been on a school trip to Germany when I was 15 and loved everything about the country. I also thought I was a bit of a native speaker, although in reality my German was 'nicht sehr gut'! So, when they told me about the 3rd Regiment Royal Horse Artillery, which had barracks in Hohne in Germany, and that they also had a decent football team, my interest was piqued. I put that down as my first choice. However, my decision changed, as

I will explain later.

I remember turning up at the Army Training Centre in Pirbright as an 18-year-old back in May 2006. It was quite a surreal feeling. Back home, I thought I was a bad boy – but all that was about to change. In reality, I was a little punk who needed all the discipline they could dish out. Surprisingly, I wasn't feeling nervous; it was almost like this was something I needed to do in order to sort myself out. If I hadn't made the decision to join the army, I would've headed down a path of working in a factory during the week, accompanied by binge drinking and taking drugs on the weekend. I knew deep down that I had more to offer and felt that I had the determination to pass the basic training and forge a successful career within the military. I decided to use the death of my mum, along with all the other pitfalls that I had experienced in my life up to now, to fuel me through the training.

The 14-week basic training course felt pretty brutal for me, in all honesty. A shock to the system, you could say. Not so much in a physical sense, as I already had a solid foundation of fitness in place thanks to football and bodybuilding, but much more in a mental sense. The lack of guidance throughout my childhood meant I had to figure things out for myself, so the 14-week training helped my self-esteem grow significantly.

I hadn't really been taught many life skills by those older than me as I grew up. Before I joined the army, I was accountable to no one. I could stay out drinking all night and no one could tell me otherwise. My life often consisted of playing football and video games, rather than trying to improve my social skills. It all seemed pretty cool at the time, but I had no real life experience or purpose to show for it. Many of my friends had family they could gain wisdom from or speak to for advice, but I was on my own. I didn't help myself, either. I didn't make much effort trying to improve my situation; instead, I resorted to the idea that I wouldn't amount to much.

The demon that already destroyed my family, alcohol, would temporarily take my pain away and distract me from my distorted reality. Before I joined the army, I had several different jobs. Some lasted longer than others, but one day I would just not show up for work; back then I was lazy and felt that life should be given to me on a plate. Classic victim mentality. The thought of waking up at 6:30 in the winter to catch a bus in order to earn £50 a day meant that I was going nowhere with that attitude. You must be shaking your head, thinking, "Welcome to the real world!" but I thought everything would be set up for me on a plate after all my hardships. Truth is, life isn't fair and no one owes you anything. Harsh, I know, but true.

I recall meeting up with a support worker named Ginny. She created a lot of job openings and courses for me to go on. However, I always said yes only to appease her. I then either backed out at the last minute or didn't turn up. I must have been a nightmare to mentor and it was a comment she made that was a reality check. She said I needed to go out and get more life experience. I'm not really sure why it struck a chord with me so much, but that was just what I needed. I realised that partying was pretty much useless when it came to building a life and a future for myself.

Finding a mentor, whether it is for work, fitness or life, can be of huge benefit. Having a coach or mentor who has the necessary skills and experience that you don't currently have can massively increase your chances of success.

I had always had a way of letting myself talk myself out of things. It was now time to stop the excuses and take action.

During my basic training, I made some great friends who I still keep in close contact with today. One of my best friends is Tom. We have good memories of basic training together and of our time later when we joined the 29th Commando Regiment Royal Artillery.

Getting the wake-up call at six in the morning was pretty tough to start with. More so after being this person who didn't see the pleasure in getting up some days. I enjoyed the physical training aspect of basic training; however, towards the end of the course I remember injuring my knee and limping for a while. I had to fight through the pain in order to be able to pass out with my troop. My determination and physical ability shone through and my troop commander, Captain Tom Sawyer (who, in January 2011, was killed in Afghanistan as one of my regiment 29 Commando members), said that I was going to a specialist regiment. For me, that meant either 29 Commando Regiment or 7 Parachute Regiment Royal Horse Artillery. I'm not sure why 29 stuck out for me, but it was the best decision I made after joining the army in the first place. I thank my troop commander for giving me the opportunity to go to 29 Commando and attempt the All Arms Commando Course to earn the coveted green beret.

Incidentally, I was recently walking back to the car with Reggie after watching a football match at Watford's Vicarage Road stadium. This was in the early stages of the break up with Roxy and I was going through a really tough time. It was then that I saw, by sheer coincidence, a road sign for 'Thomas Sawyer Way'. That inspired me to get out of the low mood I was currently in. I believe the universe is sending us signals every day, be it song lyrics, a book title… it's out there and it is up to us to find it.

Going into 29 Commando meant I had to work on my fitness and other military skills even more if I was to even think about passing the arduous All Arms Commando Course. This was to be the next goal on my journey once I had arrived at the regiment. Before that, I had to pass the basic training phase one and two, then pass a pre-commando course after that! I was glad that my hard work was rewarded at the end of phase one training. At the passing out parade, I received the Soldier's Soldier Medal, which was awarded to the recruits that my peers on the course perceived as the most worthy of it. My aim was not only to get through the basic training, but also to help everyone else on the course to pass. I have never been one for confrontation, so when I saw lads fighting and arguing, I felt a surge of responsibility to reason with them and was known as a bit of a Jack Russell when I got going!

Once we'd finished the basic training, we were sent to the Royal School of Artillery in Larkhill to do what is known as trade training. For me, this meant learning how to use the L118 light gun, which was used by 29 Commando on exercises around the world such as in Norway and on operations in Afghanistan. All of which I would get the chance to experience in due course.

Welcome to Plymouth

My first experience of Plymouth and 29 Commando didn't quite go according to plan. It was a dark, cold Sunday evening in December. I remember getting off the train from Bristol to Plymouth at about 8pm. Carrying my two big black army grips (holdalls) containing all my equipment, I hailed one of the black Hackney cabs that were waiting outside the station. I put the bags in the back and walked around to jump into the passenger side when, to my shock and disbelief, the cab driver drove off!

I had always been told to keep my wits about me when out and about in a new city, but the thought that I had been robbed of all my army kit before I even arrived sent me into sheer panic mode. I tried chasing down the cab, to no avail. I ran after it for about 200 metres or so before it sped away into the distance. So I got my phone out and called the local police station for help. Thankfully they managed to track down the taxi driver after contacting my new regiment, who kindly informed them that a black cab was waiting outside the gates of the Royal Citadel with no passenger. The cab driver hadn't noticed that I wasn't in the back!

An arrangement was made for him to head back to the station to pick me up. I made my way back and waited with my tail between my legs, feeling slightly embarrassed. When he arrived, the cab driver said: "I thought you were already in the back and I know you guys normally get your heads down when you're in here."

I hadn't realised that 29 was not the only regiment or part of the military based in Plymouth. The Marines and the Navy were here as well – which explains why there were a lot of people like me with big black grips at the railway station. What topped it off was that the cab driver charged me twice for the fare! However, I learned a lesson from this: don't drop your bags into a cab and then go to get in from the other side!

The Royal Citadel was a beautiful but intimidating place steeped in history. As a non-commando trained soldier preparing for the commando course, you didn't necessarily appreciate it in all its full glory, as a lot of the time you were being 'beasted' around it! This consisted of running around the battlements or touching every blue door in camp – and believe me, there must be over a hundred of these! Plenty of push ups, uphill sprints, anything to get your lungs burning! To start with I was treated like crap there, but, ironically, I enjoyed this. I felt that I needed to earn the right to be there and the only way I could do that was by being awarded the coveted green beret, which proved elusive to so many. Thankfully, for those going through training now and attached soldiers from other regiments, such as medics and clerks, times have changed and you are treated with a lot more respect. After all, you are attempting to become a future member of this prestigious regiment.

On my first night I was placed in a transit room with about five other lads and guided to a bottom bunk bed, or pit space, as it was usually known. Lads were not saying much, busy squaring their kit away. By this, I mean checking and packing their exercise kit, ironing their uniform, etc. There was a sombre mood in the room that night and I could sense a nervous energy. I found out it was because some of us would be taken to Okehampton the next day for the pre-commando training course. I was told not to unpack too much because if I was fit then I would most likely be going as well. They wanted to see green berets walking around camp rather than blue berets, and I couldn't blame them.

The Citadel is situated a stone's throw from the city centre, which offered many shopping delights and a decent night out most of the time. It was pretty comfortable staying at the Royal Citadel, as you had the evenings to yourself to go out drinking and eating in the vast array of takeaways and restaurants; you could do anything you liked, really. Some recruits had girlfriends who were local to the city too. All this was doing was softening us up rather than toughening us up, which, ultimately, was needed to pass this arduous course.

I had heard horror stories about Okehampton and some of the beastings that took place there. The camp was a former prisoner-of-war camp during the Second World War and some of the cells were still present in the back of the guardroom. The hill leading up to camp was approximately a mile long of bending steep inclines that even cars had trouble going up at times. Being in the camp at the top of this hill meant you were really exposed to the elements. That included gale force winds and rain, lots of it!

At the back of the camp was a public gateway leading to Dartmoor, which is a beautiful area, albeit with its own weather system. I recall one time it snowed in June! This place was perfect for training potential commando soldiers and improving survival skills. Each individual I had spoken to prior to arriving here told tales that sounded more horrific than the last. I realise that I too have been guilty of telling stories like these to those yet to take on the training course. We have a human tendency to make our own stories sound worse than the situation actually was at the time in order to seek validation. It is our own ego that usually takes over to improve our self-image.

That's not to say it wasn't tough because it was extremely tough! Living and training in Okehampton will humble you, for sure. Being cold and wet and running up a lot of hills were big parts of the average day in the life of a potential commando. Not to forget being shouted at and continuously assessed to see whether you would break or not. All this was done to see if you had what it takes to be put forward with the potential of passing the commando course, or if you would voluntarily withdraw under the conditions of being cold, wet and physically and mentally drained

Sadistic as it sounds, I actually enjoyed being at Okehampton. The lack of home comforts and fewer distractions allowed me to focus on pursuing my goal of getting my green beret. It puts you in a sort of a mediaeval mindset; the surroundings were a constant reminder that there would be suffering and this was not something that would be easy, but it would be worth it come the end of the 30-miler.

Earning My Green Beret

I finally arrived at Commando Training Centre in Lympstone. One step closer to the goal I was aiming for since the end of basic training. However, this was the biggest challenge so far, as the intensity of the training got more difficult each week, and more and more soldiers dropped out. Now it was constant testing. It was not so much being shouted at constantly though; you were taught what the standards were, and if you failed to pay attention to what you had been taught then you would suffer the consequences. It was down to each individual to get through the course by passing all the tests, which were staggered throughout the nine-weeks.

For those who have been to Lympstone, it is an intimidating place, not helped by the hench Royal Marines instructors, where a thrashing is a regular occurrence! I'm not just talking about the physical side, but also the mental aspect that comes with it. For example, while carrying out a fitness test, a Royal Marine physical training instructor shouting in your ear, "You've already failed!" and "Quit now!" was part of the mind games being used. Over time, depending on what state they were in, this tipped some of the soldiers over the edge, leading them to voluntarily withdraw from the course.

I decided not to drink alcohol for the duration of the course. I felt that this would only derail my fitness and, with my past troubles with alcohol, it wasn't worth the risk.

There were a lot of other people who were physically fitter than I was, so they could get away with having a few drinks whereas I knew that I would struggle. About halfway through the course some lads decided to go out for the night in Exmouth. I politely declined, and I'm glad I did as apparently it turned into a bit of a late night and I know that one or two of the lads that were out that night subsequently failed the six-mile weighted booted run the following Monday. This meant they would get squadded back to week one.

During this time, I also couldn't afford to eat too much junk food because a lot of the tests involved lifting your own body weight, plus 21 pounds and a standard SA80 issued rifle on your back! Climbing up a 30-foot rope or over the obstacles around the Tarzan assault course while carrying this weight make it challenging, and I didn't need to carry any extra to weigh me down. What worried me most on the course, of all things, was the 6-foot wall on the assault course! Being only 5 foot 4 inches, I struggled to climb this bad boy, especially with the 21 pounds and a rifle weighing me down. For that reason, I decided I had to go down on an evening and practice climbing the wall, much to the amusement of my colleagues.

Looking back, sometimes you have to use your own time to work on your weaknesses and do uncomfortable things like this in order to achieve the desired outcomes.

The advantages of being small in stature did have an upside. It meant that tests such as the endurance course, where you have to crawl through what is known as the Smartie tubes – two small concrete tubes, around ten metres in length – with all your kit on was much easier for someone my size! Not to forget the infamous sheep dip, where you are pushed through a tunnel under water and grabbed by someone else at the other end. It was made famous by the 2001 Royal Marines advert and struck fear in those who had not attempted it before. Something else that I had a slight advantage in most of the time was the 200-metre fireman's carry test, which is completed within 90 seconds as part of the bottom field pass out. Being a smaller person, you can feel like the most wanted person in the world when the instructors tell the course to pick a partner to carry! I'm usually around about 68 kg so when someone potentially a foot taller and an extra 20kg heavier grabs hold of me, it felt almost impossible for me to carry them, whereas carrying me would feel like a walk in the park.

I was quite fortunate that smartphones were in their infancy at the time. It would have been another unnecessary distraction on my quest to pass one of the toughest courses in the military. To this day, mobile devices mean we are more distracted and connected than ever. The latest mobile phones are incredible devices that dictate much of our lives, to the extent that we almost can't live without them. I feel that this state of being constantly connected puts us on a constant state of alert. When you have finished your contracted work hours, there are still opportunities for you to be called by your boss or to check your emails. This never-ending link prevents us from fully relaxing and switching off from the world.

I put an app blocker on my phone during the day, meaning I cannot access social media in my work hours. My notifications are also on silent to limit distractions. We all know that once you scroll at one thing it tends to lead to another and another.

How many times do you see people walking down the

street staring at a screen, seemingly totally oblivious to what's going on around them? It seems like we're losing our attention span, we struggle to focus and we are not living in the present moment. I feel we are all guilty of this from time to time. We look online to seek validation from others, when the people you should be seeking validation from are the ones sitting in the same room as you.

As I was going through the nine weeks of the commando course, the military action taking place in Afghanistan never crossed my mind. However, it would be almost inevitable that I would be deployed there not long after the course. It was not something that was really spoken about at that time, as our main focus was more centred on thoughts such as, "How many miles is the endurance course?" or "What is the first bit of scran you will eat once this is over?" We fantasised about junk food a lot while on the exercise; it took our minds off the cold and wet, accompanied by repetitive ration packs.

I remembered visualising myself getting through each test one at a time. Whenever I had five minutes to spare, I pictured myself crossing the finish line of each test. All I cared about was getting through each one and being handed my green beret at the end of the 30-miler, the final test. This meant sacrificing certain things, like going out with friends, or eating to excess, in my case. The visualisation definitely helped me and I feel it is worth investing time in doing this, especially before a big event. Try doing this for ten minutes a day. Some days you will get nothing out of it but then other times your self-conscious mind will kick in and bring more clarity to what it is you want and how you will get it. Try to conjure up as many little details as you can in your mind, from the location to who else will be there, what emotions you will be feeling and what senses you can feel. What positive outcomes will happen and what obstacles can stop you before the event? If you've already been to the location before or somewhere similar, can you use those senses you experienced, such as certain smells?

Looking back on the All Arms Commando Course, there were some parts that were very enjoyable, as it pushes you to your limits and helps you grow as a person. It is extremely tough and with that comes suffering and pushing boundaries of your previous capabilities. Once you are pushed to that level of pain, both physically and mentally, you know there is nothing you can't achieve. There are several times when you feel like you want to quit when you are on exercise, cold and wet with a lack of sleep added on top. The option of quitting with the lure of going back to a nice warm bed is always there, and the mind wants you to seek safety. But for me, I never wanted to voluntarily withdraw, mainly because I didn't want to let any of my fellow course members down.

I remember when people quit, it had repercussions. For example, we would have to assume the role of that person, either by carrying more equipment or competing against other sections that had more people in them. From the ejected look on the faces of some of the people who quit, it seemed it was at first a relief, shortly followed by them regretting the decision.

My aim was to take it day by day and prepare for each test as best as I could. I'd always thought I was pretty good at running because of my years of training beforehand, but carrying the heavy weight in our bergans (rucksacks), which we did regularly as commandos, meant I sometimes struggled keeping up because of my short foot strides! The

Tarzan assault course was a struggle because of my height, but there were shorter people than me who had passed the course in the past, so it was all possible, I told myself. It was just me in my head, looking for excuses for why I couldn't do something.

The hard work and determination paid off, as I crossed the finish line of the 30-miler and earned the right to wear the green beret. This was a very proud moment for me and showed me that I am not a quitter. It gave me a new-found confidence that had been missing for large chunks of my life. I returned to the Royal Citadel with my head held high, thinking that I now had what it took to belong there. Which I did – although I was now bottom of the pile and treated that way at first! This meant I would have to work my way up through the ranks with time served and by showing excellent performance – much like I did during the commando course. Some lads would ease off their physical training once they got into the regiment, but I had always wanted to stay prepared for the challenges that came my way.

When times got tough, I would think back to the roots of why I started this. For me, it was a combination of my troubled upbringing, proving all the doubters wrong, and my late troop commander putting his faith in me that I would pass this course and be a good fit for the regiment. As I went through phase two training, there was an elusiveness surrounding the regiment that appealed to me and made it stand out even more from the others.

The physical aspects were gruelling but also something that I enjoyed; besides, I didn't want to look back with any regrets of not trying. I have heard that passing the commando course requires the same level of fitness as an

Olympic athlete; it makes you part of the one percent of fittest people in the world. I was happy to take that honour, but that wasn't the aim I had in mind. It wouldn't be too long until my next challenge was to arrive.

Operation Herrick 9

Following the invasion of Afghanistan by the US and UK military in 2001, and me now passing the commando course, it almost seemed inevitable that I would be deployed here sooner rather than later. It was something I was looking forward to. Now a part of the Elite 3 Commando Brigade, I went out there with my regiment in October 2008. People told me the winters were really harsh out there, but during that month it was still hotter than the British summer so we had to acclimatise!

After passing the commando course, it was straight into six months of pre-deployment training to get ready for the challenges that Operation Herrick had to offer. It was quite a scary and surreal moment, the thought of deploying to what was arguably the most dangerous country in the world. It's one of the main reasons why you join up, plus you don't want to let any of your comrades down. You build up close friendships during your service and the camaraderie in the military is second to none. Even in a war zone, cheerfulness under adversity and a dark sense of humour is needed to help get you through some of the toughest days.

I guess you could put it down to the fear of the unknown, along with that underlying feeling of not coming back alive. I imagine it must play at the back of everyone's minds, the 'what if?' It gave me a sense of purpose and pride in knowing that I was playing my part in protecting and making the UK a safer place to live.

I don't really talk too much about my time in Afghanistan. I don't think a lot of soldiers do. I remember coming back and always having the same questions fired at me, like "How many people have you killed?" and "Have you been shot at yet?" As you can imagine, these are very personal and invasive questions and I'm not quite sure what response they are looking for.

That is one of the main reasons that I don't speak much about it. The other reason is that one of the briefs we were given ahead of our return to the UK was along the lines of "You can tell your friends and family about some of the scenes you witnessed out there, but they won't be able to truly comprehend it as much as you do, and some people won't even care what you've done!" I think it's human nature to talk about ourselves highly and even show off when given the opportunity. This isn't me. I downplayed any conversations about Afghanistan and didn't really talk about it unless I was with my fellow comrades.

When you are out there for so long, you have to try and detach yourself by not thinking about loved ones back home. As selfish as it sounds, you have to put it to the back of your mind temporarily, otherwise it will break you down mentally. Plus, if you are in a war zone and your mind is on something else then you could be in trouble. I was with my first wife at the time; this was before my eldest boy Reggie had been born. I'm sure it would have been even tougher being out there and leaving my child. I'm not sure how some of the others who had children got through the whole tour being without them for so long. We had satellite phones that could be used to call loved ones back home, along with 30 minutes a week on a card that could be topped up when needed, so it wasn't all bad.

Arriving at Camp Bastion for the first time was definitely eye-opening. The UK and US bases were huge, and one of the biggest shocks was seeing a KFC and Pizza Hut out in the middle of the desert! Not that I ate at either of them as they were closed a lot of the time. It didn't appeal to me too much, and I had my protein powder to keep me going instead.

About a week later, we flew out of Camp Bastion to a city towards the north of Helmand Province called Musa Qala. We had overtaken the previous artillery regiment that were operating the three L118 light guns out of an FOB (Forward Operating Base) that was providing fire support to the marines and members of our regiment who were out on the ground as fire support teams. The L118 light gun is an amazing weapon used in operations around the world, from the Falklands to the Middle East, as well in as the extreme cold of Norway. To clarify, despite what the name might suggest, it weighs around 1600kg so it is definitely not light, but smaller and more manoeuvrable than most other artillery weapons.

Once we were acquainted with the FOB, I was pleased to realise that there was a half decent gym. This helped keep me occupied throughout our time there. It's also true that in our downtime we did a lot of sunbathing! A common occurrence during that tour was when we were called to carry out a fire mission. It was a race against time to run back from the gym or wherever we were to put on our body armour and man the guns ready to fire. Every second counted for the allies that needed our support in the thick of the action. We spent the tour with an Australian artillery regiment, who were a great bunch of guys and helped to keep the morale high throughout the tour.

It was a combination of lots of downtime, followed by manning the guns and firing hundreds of high-explosive rounds up to a distance of 17.2km for what could be several hours a day at a time. It was an eye-opening experience for sure. Being in danger and spending so long away from home strengthened my armour and developed my resilience. I believe that going through the adversity I encountered in my earlier years helped me to cope out there and adapt my mindset fairly quickly. I was used to the feeling of being alone and going through hard times.

Upon my return to the UK I enjoyed a well-deserved six weeks off to reintegrate with society. However, it wouldn't be too long until I was back out there again.

Operation Herrick 14

Only two years later, in 2011, and we were back out in Afghanistan again. You could almost call me a veteran of the place by now! Only kidding, but it felt great to be able to pass on my knowledge to the younger members who had joined since that first tour and I felt good about teaching others. It was the first sign that teaching was something I really enjoyed and possibly wanted to do after a career in the military.

This second tour was a whole lot different to the first. By this stage of the war the light guns were not really used, possibly because of the collateral damage they caused. Instead, we were trying to plan our exit from the country and win the hearts and minds of the locals.

This meant that instead of sitting around not doing much during these six months, the opportunity came about to move to a more hostile area into an infantry role, which meant going out on foot patrols each day and getting up close and personal with the Taliban as well as local villagers. This was something that was terrifying at first, but you had to adapt quickly to these situations and there was no room for error. Our role was to make our presence known in the local areas and gain intel on any senior Taliban leaders who were operating in the area. Out of respect for all those I served with, and as I mentioned earlier, it is best not to go into too much detail, but let's just say the adrenaline was extreme and it is something that will stick in my mind for the rest of my life.

One of the areas we controlled was split into three different checkpoints, which were small areas, maybe one or two compounds big and as close to the Taliban as you could get. In the morning there was evidence that they had been outside and at times they even tried to scale the walls to gain access! We were vastly outnumbered when we stayed at these checkpoints but felt that we always had enough firepower to get out of there if we were under attack. Another critical aspect was that we all had faith in each other that we were highly trained and had each other's backs.

When out on patrol, we spoke to the locals in the area, who would sometimes invite us into their homes. The women and children stayed out of the way in a separate room, which is how the culture is over there. We were often offered chai (tea) once inside. There was one occasion when I could've sworn there was more than just chai in that cup! Understandably, for the safety of their family they were very tight-lipped about whether there were any Taliban in the area, as the Taliban could pay them a visit during the night under the cover of darkness when we were most likely back at our checkpoints.

I'm not sure the exact weights of the daysacks we carried, but with all the ammunition, water etc., it could be anywhere in excess of 30kg, plus I had a general-purpose machine gun and ammunition with me that weighed another 20kg! You can imagine trying to patrol with all this in temperatures of up to 50 degrees. You need to have a lot of determination, grit and will to keep going or the consequences could mean death if you come under attack or get heatstroke from the searing temperatures.

We set up a checkpoint in an abandoned school that was on top of a large hill, of all places! By all accounts the school was built for the village children but then never used. Our section of seven set up home in one of the classrooms, which was equipped with a blackboard. The benefit of our new checkpoint being on top of a hill was that we had a great vantage point looking over the whole area.

I am always amazed when visiting different countries and seeing other cultures. They say travel broadens the mind, and for me it allows me to empathise more with people and experience different perspectives. We don't know what somebody is going through, so all we can do is try to see the situation from their point of view. I had a strong feeling that the villagers didn't really want us there. They were tired from many years of suffering under the Taliban. It seemed that even though we were trying to protect them, us being around made their lives that bit more stressful.

The little kids would pester us a lot for anything they could get their hands on. Whether it was pens or melted chocolate, they wanted to trade it with us. In exchange, we wanted the delicious pomegranate fruit that grew on the trees. Their bartering skills got better over time: it started with just one chocolate bar for a piece of fruit, which then turned into two or sometimes three bars! Chocolate melted from the heat was almost useless for us, but an unknown and delicious treat not always experienced by the children. They also traded Afghan foot bread, which was amazing. Some of the best bread that I've had. Either that, or I had been away too long by that point!

While I was in Afghanistan, along with the north east African country of Djibouti, I went to some of the poorest areas that I visited during my time in the army. What surprised me was that despite not having a lot, and the desolate conditions, the people still laughed and joked. There were no material possessions or comparisons with one another; they were just grateful with what they had and made a decision to make the most of it.

One thing I and many of my colleagues found ourselves doing during tours was counting down the days until we were back home. Looking back, that seems crazy: life is short enough as it is, so to just wish six months of it away at a time seems like a waste of time, literally. Once that time is gone, you're not getting it back.

I had a great experience on both tours and I am glad that it opened my eyes to some of the horrors that people all over the world are surviving on a daily basis. The point I'm trying to make here is that I was not using those days to try and make them more productive to improve myself. On a personal level, this included planning for my future. That's not to say we weren't busy, but there was also a lot of downtime. I saw a few guys out there who were studying for an online degree. They had a plan in place that they wanted to leave the military when they got back. They were improving their professional development in order to increase the chances of employment once on civilian street. This made me question my own choices; I wasn't going to spend my whole career in the army (and, unfortunately, my career ended a bit sooner than I hoped because of my illness), but if you are always learning, you are always growing as a person. Education shouldn't stop at school, that's for sure. It needs to be a lifelong journey leading to fulfilment and, ultimately, it is one of the reasons to feel in a state of happiness.

I decided that once I got back, I would invest a lot more in my personal development – initially as a back-up plan, but it turned out I would need it sooner than anticipated.

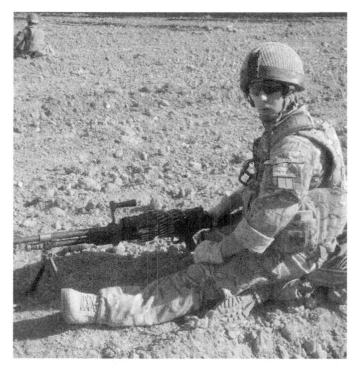

Operation Herrick 14

Norway

Another big part of being a commando includes being able to operate in all weather climates around the world. One such place is the beautiful but extremely cold country of Norway. The training was usually located to the north of the country, where temperatures are a lot harsher. Therefore, this makes the training and survival phases all the more challenging, thus adding another level of strength to my armour, you could say, to add to my unbreakable resilience.

The lowest temperatures we faced during my two visits to Norway were up to minus 50 degrees with the wind chill! Usually, all training ceases if the temperature reaches minus 30, so when this did happen, we were ordered into our vehicles to try and escape the potentially fatal conditions.

Training in these conditions is not to be taken lightly. If an individual is not on top of their game and personal admin, the consequences can be catastrophic. Frostnip, which I had in my right index finger, can lead to frostbite of the extremities, hypothermia and – worst case scenario – death. Then there are several other hazards, such as dehydration, injuring yourself while skiing and even falling through the ice!

Fortunately, the instructors, who were Royal Marines mountain leaders, are a different breed from the rest of us. Highly trained via an arduous course to become a mountain leader and be able to lead others in treacherous conditions, it means that if things go wrong, they know what to do!

My deployment here was broken down into three main phases. First, I had to complete survival week. This was required for all those who wanted to be able to leave camp, which was granted in the limited downtime we had in between exercises. It provided you with some of the necessary skills needed in case you were outside camp and got into difficulty with the unpredictable weather. This phase consisted of five days learning how to ski with full kit on, spending four of these nights sleeping out. One of them involved digging for several hours in order to build a quinzee for our section of up to eight people to sleep in. In layman's terms, this is a snow shelter constructed from loose snow, then shaped and hollowed out so we could access and egress this enormous snow pile. It was big enough to fit us all in and had sleep shelves where we spent the night. Ironically, I felt warmer that night than in the tent! We poked an oxygen hole through the ceiling so we didn't suffer asphyxiation and took part in what is known as 'candle watch', where we took turns staying awake to check the flame was still burning, indicating that the hole was still allowing oxygen to be present in the quinzee.

The final day of this short but very sharp survival week was topped off with what is known as ice breaker drills. Not quite sitting in a warm, comfortable classroom talking about yourself to others, but more simulating a potential incident of falling through the frozen ice while skiing with your kit on! For this, a ginormous block of ice was drilled out of a frozen lake, leaving an ice-cold pool approximately two metres wide and three metres long. One by one, you're invited to slip on a pair of skis, then unbuckled and tied to a rope, so you can be slipped off and pulled back in by the instructors. From there, a rope tied like a lasso is put around your head and under one of your armpits in order to pull you out in case you can't get back out or disappear under the ice. To top this off, you put a bergen on one shoulder filled with a 20kg jerry can of water, although ours would've been considerably heavier with our full kit and weapon. Once you slip on the skis and bergen, you are handed a pair of ski poles, which are held in one hand to reduce the chance of dropping one. Once you are ready, the plan is to slide into the baltic water, control your breathing, pull your bergen out of the water first and make your way back to the edge. Once you have calmed your breathing again and stuck the sharp edges of the ski poles into the ice like daggers, there is a requirement to shout your number, rank and name to the instructor to gain permission to get out of the water! From this point, it is sheer grit in order to keep digging those ski poles in and pulling yourself out. All this while everyone is watching you! The final part of this evolution concludes with rolling around in the snow, accompanied by drinking a shot of something strong. What, I can't remember; rum or brandy, possibly.

Once free to grab your kit, you go into a large tent with a roaring heater. The aim is to get changed as quickly as possible, despite your fingers feeling like they are on fire!

Cold water immersion is a popular habit among elite athletes, as well as everyday people, for its amazing benefits. I know we don't always have a freezing lake available, so the most common way of achieving this is through cold showers, or even more extreme in the form of ice baths! Some of the benefits include reducing stress, building up resilience and exercise recovery, and it also boosts your immune system and circulation.

With survival week completed, the second part of the

novice course included a manoeuvre week. This involves donning skis, or, if in difficult areas, ski shoes, and conducting long distance moves across the training areas with a troop of around 40-50 people. All this while carrying full exercise kit and rifles. If by this stage you hadn't mastered how to ski properly, doing it while carrying heavy equipment meant you were in for a lot of suffering! The constant falling down and trying to get up again with 30kg plus of equipment while wearing skis... one can only imagine how draining this is on your energy and morale. It also had a knock-on effect on the other members of the troop. Having to wait for the slower skiers meant a lot of waiting around getting cold, with the heavy kit digging into your back and shoulders. The longer each move took, the less time was available to set up our tents and get our heads down for the night and recover, but we never left anyone behind.

This week was the one in particular that required a lot of grit and resilience to keep on going and push through pain barriers, while helping other members of your eight-man section in the process. But when the tent was finally set up, there was no time to rest. There were several jobs that needed doing, like boiling lots of hot water to cook our meals and make hot drinks with, refilling the snow peak stoves and lamp with kerosene oil, and personal admin such as drying any clothing and maintaining a watch rota to ensure the lamp didn't go out and release poisonous carbon monoxide while everyone slept.

The third and final week of the novice course was the tactics and manoeuvre phase. Slightly more brutal – but as some improvements had been made in skiing, it didn't feel quite so draining in that sense. However, carrying out section attacks in knee-deep snow can get pretty emotional and your lungs burn from running in snowshoes with kit on! I don't have as many memories of that week – just that it was painful, and that I knew it was the final phase to get through in order to finish the training. I do remember the course ending with a long ski/walk for several miles to where the lovely warm transport was waiting to pick us up. A time limit was placed on getting there and if the directing staff checked your flask and it was not full of hot liquid, chances were you could fail the whole course!

I felt so much relief when this training was over. Some liken it to the All Arms Commando Course, only shorter. There is also a requirement to stay up to date by completing it every five years. My first trip was in 2008 and my second trip fell in 2013, meaning that I had just run out so I was ordered to do two courses of suffering! Putting all this aside, the suffering was worth it in order to appreciate this beautiful country even more.

Leaving the Military

All good things must come to an end, or so I've been told. I thought I was destined to serve a full 22-year career in the army. Unfortunately, it wasn't to be. The 12 years I did serve changed my life in ways I couldn't imagine. Looking back now at 18-year-old me, the 'What ifs' of not joining don't bear thinking about; I don't know where I would've ended up otherwise.

To say that my world came crashing down at this point would be an understatement. Serving in 29 Commando gave me great pride and purpose, it was a stable and steady career, plus I could get paid to have a laugh with mates and to keep fit!

I believe some soldiers can adapt to change and civilian life fairly quickly, whereas for me, it took a while because of a number of different factors. I was living with heart disease and had the added pressure of preparing for the birth of my second boy, Luca, just a few months before my medical discharge. I had this overwhelming thought in my head that no company would want to hire someone with a long-term illness and a risk of potentially dying at any moment. A classic case of me overthinking things again.

I enjoy a challenge and was determined to find a new career that would pay around the same as I had been earning in the military so our standard of living didn't change too much, especially with the new arrival on the way. There are a lot of misconceptions that employers love to employ ex-military people but that isn't always the case. Here I was at the age of 30 having never written a CV or attended a job interview in at least twelve years!

Fortunately, when I was posted at Larkhill in Salisbury for two years before I found out about the ARVC, I made the most of the opportunity to improve my professional development and gain some valuable skills and qualifications that would make my transition from the military to civilian life a little smoother. Even though I had no intention of leaving the military at that point, it is always better to be prepared for whatever life throws at you – and let's just say life threw one big sucker punch at me shortly afterwards.

I had struck up a great friendship with a man named Rob Dawkins, who was a 22-year army veteran and in charge of the Royal Artillery Continuing Professional Development (RACPD) centre. Rob was extremely helpful in researching options and finding out what funding was available for me to undertake courses I was interested in. In return, I think he appreciated my drive and determination to work hard to complete these courses.

That's when it started for me: the realisation that even if I had a 22-year military career, I would still only be 40 years old. Potentially, I still had another 20 years or so to work until pension age, never mind other factors out of my control, such as redundancies – which I swerved once or twice – or even falling out of love with the military and seeking a new career closer to home.

I researched what courses I could study that would benefit my current role, such as management or health and safety, as well as courses I could study at night. I also made a list of things I enjoyed doing as a kid, which mostly consisted of playing football, gym or computer games. Although you can have a very successful career in these areas in this day and age, I had to refine it slightly to suit my personality and style of learning. I enjoyed problem solving, attention to detail, working on my own or as part of a team. The opportunity came up for some courses relating to health and safety, so I took them and ended up enjoying it, and that is the career I am doing today. I know it may be some people's idea of hell, but we all have different ways of working and finding where we can provide value for others.

It was all well and good having these qualifications to my name, but with no experience to back it up, along with my low self-esteem back again in full swing, it became my aim to find a rewarding new career while preparing for my medical discharge from the army.

I had to sit on an army medical board, which consisted of both military and civilian doctors who assessed my medical history and would ultimately decide if I would be able to fulfil the needs of the army in years to come. I didn't hold too much hope because a soldier who is deployed on exercises or operations at home and abroad has to be physically fit and healthy, something I wasn't necessarily going to be in the long run. As I had the ICD embedded in my chest, holding metal or any type of electromagnetic charge could react with it and set it off. Besides, if I fell ill in the middle of nowhere, trying to get me to a cardiologist quickly would be an extremely difficult task. I hoped I would be able to carry out a desk role somewhere so I could still sense that feeling of pride that comes with being in the army.

Just after my 31st birthday, in June 2018, the date was

set for me to become a civilian again. If you ask me if I had fully transitioned since that point, the answer is probably no. However, I did have a solid nine months of uninterrupted employment in my first role since leaving the forces, until February 2019 when things started to decline.

This is when I experienced the first bouts of ventricular tachycardia, the rapid, irregular heartbeat that can make you struggle to breathe. The worrying thing about this horrible disease is that it can show its presence at any point. For me, it always seemed to be on a Friday night! I remember some of the Friday nights we would spend in the back of an ambulance travelling to hospital through the centre of Bristol, with drunk party goers banging on the back trying to get in. "Oh, how I wish I could have nights like that again where I am carefree and can enjoy myself," I thought quietly to myself.

Over the next few months my heart got progressively worse. Having what was once talked about as a condition I could live with for the rest of my life, to being told that a heart transplant is the only option left for you, definitely puts things into perspective.

Worse still, my cardiologist at the time gave me the news that the average life expectancy of a heart transplant patient is 10 years. That would mean I could be dead by 42; my boys would only be 10 and 16! (I believe this figure of 10 years is based on an average, as there are now heart transplant patients enjoying up to 35 extra years after their operation, and maybe even meeting the criteria to have a second heart transplant!)

By this time, I was working about two hours a day until gradually that became too much for me. Normal everyday tasks such as walking the dogs and cooking were a challenge. Since the first episode of VT back in February, I had surrendered my driving licence, so I had to rely on Roxy to transport me to and from work and hospital appointments.

We went on a family holiday to Newquay in November as a replacement for the honeymoon we had booked to Costa Rica, which I was in no fit state to travel to! Newquay was our next best option, and even then, we cut the holiday short by three days as I wasn't feeling great and was quite limited in what I could do.

In the space of 18 months, my priorities had shifted from having a successful career with which I could afford a family home, to staying alive long enough for the call that a heart was available. But whatever came at me, I wasn't going down without a fight. I had got through all the challenges in life so far, and I believed it wasn't my time to go yet.

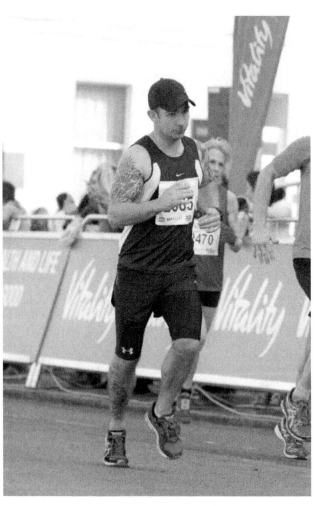

March 2016: This was taken only four months before the irregular heart beat was discovered and at a time when I felt on top of the world

.

Part III
Life After Transplant

The Two Weeks After Transplant

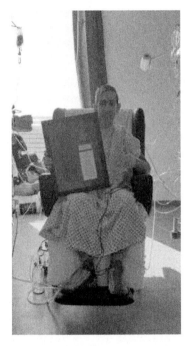

*April 2020: I had finally made it! Even though
I was in a lot of pain when this photo was taken,
I felt like the happiest person alive.*

I made it!

The operation had been a huge success, so I was told. I vividly remember waking up after surgery feeling like I had been hit by a bus. Every movement I attempted was sheer agony, but I had done it! It was worth this intense pain, which would slowly subside over the coming days and weeks.

It was early evening by the time I woke up, roughly about 8pm, meaning the operation took around 6-8 hours to complete. Time was all a bit of a blur during that last 48 hours. It was almost over. A culmination of nearly five months in intensive care, along with the three years of struggle, dating back to March 2017 when I first found out about the heart disease, to be now given this new opportunity... There was no chance I was going to sleep that night! A combination of endorphins swimming around my brain accompanied by the throbbing pain from my sternum made getting any sleep nearly impossible.

The next day was all a bit chaotic, as lots of different doctors came in to check on my progress and carry out various tests. Some junior doctors I hadn't seen before came to visit, almost like they wanted to see a heart transplant patient for the first time after the operation. Not that I minded; I was lapping up the attention! Either that, or I was likely too tired to offer much resistance! I spent two days in the intensive care unit so they could keep an eye on me, as this was the most critical stage and they had to check that the new heart was beating well in its new home.

I was finally moved to the hallowed ward upstairs, a lot less chaotic and more relaxing than the ICU I had become accustomed to. It was a clear sign that I was progressing well. Ironic as it sounds, even though it was at the top of the building, it was a step closer to leaving the hospital and going home! It felt surreal watching the monitor I was connected to showing my new heartbeat, beating away in all its glory. It was beautiful and I stared at it for hours, thinking how proud and grateful I was. I actually had a fully beating heart in my chest again!

What was really surreal, and prevented me from sleeping at times, was hearing my own heartbeat as I lay on my side to rest. The average heart rate of a heart transplant patient is around 90-100 beats per minute and sometimes more. As you can imagine, this was a lot faster than I was used to! While I was connected to the BiVAD machine, it beat my failing heart for me at 60 beats per minute, which could be adjusted as and when required. Now here I was, marvelling at a sound I hadn't heard in such a long time! It felt deafeningly loud in my ear and I'm still getting used to this. It is a pleasant reminder at the end of each day that I am still here, beating away, and everything is alright.

I discovered a new level of gratitude from that day onwards. It has changed my perspective on life, for sure. A lot of people approached me afterwards and said that I deserved a bit of luck after what I had been through. However, from my perspective, I was one of the luckiest people alive. At the time of writing, there are currently 312 people in the UK on the waiting list for a heart transplant[2]. There are many people who don't survive long enough to receive a life-saving transplant in time. This is why organ donation is so vitally important.

Prior to the transplant, my chances of survival were minimal. One of the cardiologists told Roxy that I should've died six months before I came to Papworth! If I hadn't exercised and eaten well most of the time then I don't think my heart would've been strong enough to survive up to that

---

2   https://www.statista.com/statistics/519812/active-organ-waiting-list-united-kingdom-uk/

point. I felt, deep inside, a premonition that it wasn't my time to go yet. I still had more to offer. Although survival was out of my control, thanks to all the great staff at Papworth and my positive attitude throughout, I did survive and walked out just fourteen days later after eight operations, which involved opening up my chest three times.

My mind was uneasy at times, racing with more questions than answers. What was my donor like? How did they come to pass away? What must their family be going through having to say goodbye to their loved one? A plethora of emotions, from sadness to joy, flickered back and forth until I realised that the donor and their family would want me to make the most of this precious gift. So that is what I intended to do. Easy in theory, although mentally and physically, it is not always so easy to do. The doctors tend to explain it as trading in one set of problems for another. I had a better set of problems now though, for sure.

I was given a little blue book to list all my medications in, and wow, there were so many at first! Looking back, there must've been at least ten different types of medication, all with names that are challenging to pronounce at first try. As my condition has improved, I have been weaned off several of these medications. The main ones that I still use to this day are the anti-rejection drugs that a transplant patient takes twice a day for the rest of their life. This is because the body's natural immune system sees the new organ as a foreign object and, quite rightly, tries to fight it.

Therefore, I am now immunosuppressed, which means I am more susceptible to illness than the average person with a healthy immune system. This explains why some of the population, such as me, had to shield for a large period of time during the pandemic, because we are classed as being clinically extremely vulnerable.

Some of the other meds that I took, such as prednisolone, a corticosteroid that fights inflammation in the body, also help to defend against rejection of the new organ. They can have some horrible side effects, such as mood swings, tiredness, acne, increased appetite and giving you the appearance of a 'moon face', which I was all too paranoid about. Some patients remain on these for life, whereas others will wean off them gradually in the first year. Thankfully, I was in the latter group.

Each passing day after the transplant I was feeling stronger. The physios left an exercise bike and a stepper in my room, so, me being me, I would hop on the bike for five to ten minutes or as long as I could last several times a day to help pass the time. At first, I managed about five on each leg on the step ups because of my weak leg strength and balance. However, a week or so later, I was doing 20 each leg and getting some very odd looks from people walking past my room!

After pretty much coming back from the dead after all the operations in December and January, I had made it my mission to go for a daily walk, pushing my trolley containing the BiVAD machines, and assisted by nurses who had to hold the four tubes protruding from my stomach while I was walking. I needed a five-person crew just so I could go for a walk! Some days I could only manage a hundred metres until my machines started beeping like crazy. Other days I managed two laps of the intensive care unit, which, at a wild guess, were maybe four hundred metres each but felt like a marathon in my head! The staff explained that those who put in the walking before the transplant tend to recover quicker and I felt this helped my recovery, for sure.

Day by day I was getting less tied down by devices, such as a urinary catheter, pacing wires and a suction pump. There was a lot of fluid build-up in my chest where one of the tubes had been positioned previously. The nurses had to keep repacking gauze into the wounds where the tubes had been sticking out of my stomach, as they kept leaking every time I moved. Eventually they stopped leaking and I had a few more stitches to hold it all in place. And I now have some pretty gnarly scars on my torso!

Once the transplant team completed an echocardiogram and were happy that the heart was looking amazing, they carried out what's known as a right heart catheterization, which involves a cardiologist taking up to five tissue samples directly from the heart to check for any signs of rejection.

Another part of the sequence of going home was knowing all my medicines by heart, as well as being trusted to take them on my own. I studied that little blue book like it was going out of fashion because I was doing everything I could to get out of there as soon as possible! The only thing that was holding me up from leaving was a blood test, which showed that my levels of tacrolimus (the anti-rejection drug that I take twice a day for life) were below the required level of eight to allow me to leave. Lower than eight meant I didn't have much immunity, and with the coronavirus out there, and not too much known about it at this stage, they deemed it safer to keep me in for another 48 hours to test it again. I had spent so long here that surely another couple of days wouldn't hurt, I thought to myself. But with the finish line nearly in sight, I was itching to get back to see my boys and sleep in my own bed. "There's not much going on out there, the whole country's in lockdown!' were the cries. I wasn't planning on going out, but just being in the comfort and safety of our own home and familiar surroundings was what I craved... oh and fresh air, lots of fresh air!

Something else that we had waiting at home for us was a pile of unopened Christmas presents that were meant for the Christmas of 2019 that didn't quite happen. I felt somewhat relieved that we didn't put the tree up before I was admitted to intensive care, as it would've felt strange taking it down in April!

Finally, the blood test results came back. My tacrolimus levels were sitting at a lofty 11, meaning I was free to go! I felt a bit guilty ringing one of my best friends, Brad, to ask to be picked up three hours away from Bristol at 5pm! Always reliable, Brad was more than glad to set his way east, picking Roxy up from the bed and breakfast and getting a takeaway first before collecting me.

When they told me they were close by, two helpful nurses helped to wheel down my massive collection of clothes, puzzles, pyjamas and duvet covers that I had accumulated during my five-month stay in Papworth. After a long-awaited reunion with Roxy and Brad, we departed the hospital – after a quick photo outside what had been my home for so long. At least until my next return there only two weeks later for another right heart catheterization!

I got into bed at precisely five past midnight and it was one of those unforgettable moments I will treasure for the rest of my life. The feeling of your own bed after being in a hospital bed for five months was heavenly. There was a streetlight outside our home, lighting up the place. I hadn't seen one of those in a while!

The biggest shock, though, was when I walked up the stairs to our bedroom in one go. The last time I tried this, I had to take a break halfway up as I was so short of breath. "This is amazing," I thought to myself, "and a sign of better things to come!"

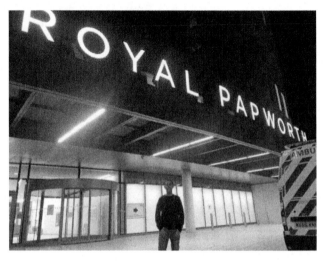

April 2020: Walking out of the place that saved my life, just two weeks later

The Rollercoaster Ride of Transplant Life

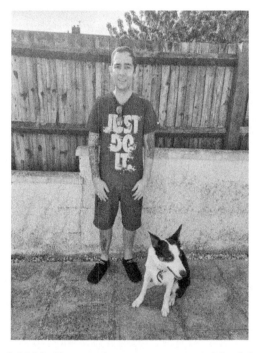

April 2020: Despite being in a national lockdown,
I was so happy to be at home with my family.

The first 12 weeks after the transplant were quite uneventful. Not only because the national lockdown was in full force, but because my sternum had been opened so many times at this point, it needed at least 12 weeks of recovery time to heal. One of the main pieces of advice you are given is not to lift heavy items during that time as you could rip open your chest! And after all that time in hospital, I didn't fancy another stint in Papworth, despite how well they had looked after me.

As well as taking the medications as prescribed, another key part of advice is to keep active daily, as light exercise can improve the function of the heart. All heart transplant patients are offered something called cardiac rehab, which basically shows patients how to exercise correctly, gradually building up their fitness. One of the main reasons for this is that during the operation, something which we all have, the vagus nerve, is detached when the old heart is removed. Also known as denervation, the vagus nerve sends signals from the brain to the heart. This explains the higher resting heart rate of 90-100 beats per minute, and it means that it's very important to warm up and cool down before exercise. The reason for this is to increase your heart rate steadily over five to ten minutes and reduce down again for the same amount of time, as this primes the body to know that exercise is about to take place. This also lets me return to a normal heart rate safely. Going all out too quickly could confuse the brain, and chances are that I would collapse. It's not happened yet, thankfully.

In some rare cases, the vagus nerve can reattach itself on its own after about five years post-transplant; there are some heart transplant patients who have gone on to compete in Ironman events! So watch this space!

The cardiac rehab was not an option for me because of the lockdown, so I had to invest in something known as a turbo trainer, a stand that a pushbike can go on in order to pedal away, making it similar to a stationary bike, which kept me entertained for a while. They were all the rage as everyone else was staying indoors and finding new ways to exercise.

Seeing my boys again was truly incredible. It was difficult that I couldn't hug them at first because other households weren't allowed to mix, and with me being classed as clinically extremely vulnerable, it made it very tough mentally. Eventually, Luca came back home after a period of isolating; then, when the restrictions were lifted, Reggie came over to stay. We had so much time to catch up, and it was amazing to see how much they had grown and developed since I last saw them properly. The way they handled being apart from me for so long during my hospital stay and the lockdown was inspirational. I know they will grow into amazing young men.

The first year after transplant is considered to be the most decisive and vulnerable. The body is still recovering after so much trauma, so mentally adapting to this 'new normal' is very tough. A heart transplant patient will attend hospital 12 times in the first year to have check-ups and further right heart catheterization. Scoring a zero following this procedure means there is no rejection and 1R shows mild rejection. 2R means the patient is in rejection and may display symptoms of swelling, breathlessness and feeling generally unwell (a bit like I did during the heart failure stage). This requires a hospital stay and some IV steroids to get rid of the rejection. Then you have 3R, which is chronic rejection. This could happen for a number of reasons: possibly someone hasn't taken the prescribed anti-rejection meds, or the kidneys or liver are not functioning as they should. They take a big hit from all the medication and this impacts the other organs, causing them issues in the future.

Thankfully, the most rejection I have had up to this date is 1R. This is fairly common while the team is trying to get the medication right, so I'm not having more than I need to and vice versa.

One of the biggest causes of death in heart transplant patients is something known as Cardiac Allograft Vascopathy (CAV). This is a narrowing of the arteries that can occur several years after transplant. It can restrict the flow of blood to the heart and lead to a heart attack or a recurrence of heart failure. I take statins to help with this, as a side effect of the anti-rejection meds can cause a furring of the arteries. See what I mean about changing one set of problems for another!

All was going as well as possible in my recovery, and I was loving being at home in the garden with my family, enjoying the great summer that we had that year. Although the old me would have been top off sunbathing, because of the low immune system I can be more prone to skin cancers, so I lather up with factor 50 sun cream, even on overcast days. The steroids were making their presence felt as I started getting acne all over my back, along with the moon face. This made me quite paranoid, even though I wasn't going out or seeing many people. Don't get me started on hair loss! I'm glad it's starting to grow back again. This is also true of my nails, as while in the hospital my nails weren't getting the nutrients and normal blood supply, eventually causing some of my toe nails to partially fall off! It took a good six months or so for those big toe nails in particular to grow back normally.

I must confess I was a little bit naughty and purchased a hot tub during the lockdown, much to the dismay of some of the transplant team! There is a risk of infection from bacteria rising up from the water, so we made sure it was as clean as possible with adequate chlorine in it. I will always be susceptible when using a public hot tub; using a private one was a safer option and I never got ill.

Our friends were a godsend before and after my transplant journey, as well as the military support charity SSAFA. They all helped to raise funds for my family and me to pay for our bills so that we had a home to go back to. Fortunately Roxy's job allowed her to work from a laptop, so while she was in hospital with me, she was also doing some work as well, when mentally able to, while I watched Netflix or slept!

My friends organised two charity events, a horse racing night and a football match, raising over £15,000 in total. Simply amazing! We will always be in their debt. Not only theirs, but the whole of our local community too. Some people I had never heard of or spoken to had been inspired by my story and wanted to help. SSAFA helped us by sending over a volunteer to visit us, a support worker named Alan, who was an RAF veteran, and we all became good friends. Alan helped to arrange a mobility scooter and storage shed to help me get around before the transplant when I was going through severe heart failure. As you can probably guess, I ended up not needing it in the end as I was in intensive care by that point! Thankfully they transferred the funds to pay our monthly bills instead. Along with SSAFA, the Royal Artillery Charitable Fund caught wind of the story and willingly donated to help us throughout this period.

All the check-ups in the first year went really well and the medical team were amazed with my progress. I had some gym weights in the garage, so, starting off really light,

I couldn't wait to get back into one of my main passions in life, bodybuilding! I had one minor – or you could say major – issue. As I mentioned before, all the nerves and muscle on my left side had been sliced through during the thoracotomy procedure. I protected it greatly for months and paid the price, as my left arm was about half the strength and size of my right arm. My first aim was to try and develop the left side of my upper body so I wasn't so out of alignment. A lot easier said than done!

My first major setback was when I got shingles about four months after transplant. I can't ever remember having chicken pox as a child and had heard stories that getting shingles as an adult can be very dangerous, even more so if you have a weakened immune system. The scabs and crusts all developed on the right side of my face, starting above my lip at first, which led my GP to think that it was impetigo. I wish! The shingles was brutal. My face became so swollen, and the nerve tingling was unbearable at times for the best part of a month. I still suffer now with post neuropathic pain in the right side of my mouth and to this day I can't chew on that side, meaning I now have to use the left side of my mouth only!

I eventually managed to get back into working out regularly at my local gym. Maybe I trained a bit too strenuously at first, or maybe it was just a case of bad luck when I noticed in the mirror one day whilst having a pee that a lump was sticking out of my stomach! I poked and prodded it. It felt soft but not painful to touch, so I visited my GP, who sent me straight to my local hospital to have a further look. After several interrogations, they couldn't fully determine what it was, as I was also feeling flu-like symptoms at the same time. Possibly a coincidence? A couple of weeks later I went to Papworth where they confirmed it to be a hernia protruding from my stomach. This can be quite common in those who have had their chests opened when they haven't fully repaired, as well as in women who have recently given birth!

The one benefit was that this meant all ab exercises were off limits, meaning I didn't have to worry so much about that ever elusive six pack! I've had to come up with other ways to work my core than endless crunches and sit ups!

A slightly more embarrassing issue, and the most troublesome of all, is my peeing problem! This was the result of having several urinary catheters inserted for so long that eventually it caused a urethra stricture, best described as scarring in the urethra tube. This makes the tube more constricted, so having a pee is very painful, plus not being able to fully empty the bladder and getting up several times during the night! Thankfully, I had an operation to fix this temporarily but it is already coming back, so a more invasive procedure is needed to cure it.

This is all a small price to pay in order to be given this second chance at life, and I am forever grateful for every day that I wake up. When I woke up while in the hospital, I kept telling myself that each day was another chance to get a heart transplant. I had a mantra from a Banksy picture that I have at home that I repeated in my head: "There is always hope." I now feel truly blessed to be spending my life with those I love, and now I want to make my donor proud, knowing that I am making the most of what I have been given.

Ever since I was a kid I have been a fan of completing tough physical challenges. After reading online and speaking to my transplant team, it turns out there is not much you can't do after receiving a new heart! I read some incredible stories about heart transplant recipients who have managed to complete Ironman competitions and I was amazed! It certainly sowed a seed. I still have that commando mentality; I needed it to get through the struggles of my hospital journey. I thought to myself: "How far can I really go?" However, I was a bit sceptical at first, as the X-rays of my left lung showed some mild cloudiness, caused by the pulmonary arrest I suffered.

I had always enjoyed running in the past. When I completed the Bristol half-marathon in 2015, I loved the buzz of being joined by thousands of other people and cheered on by hundreds on the side lines. It had a great vibe to it and I almost immediately signed up to the 2016 event, but it wasn't to be. After my bicep operation in July of that year and undergoing investigations about this potential problem, I very wisely pulled out of the race and gave my number to a friend. I felt quite gutted about it, and when the diagnosis unravelled and my condition worsened, the thought of being able to run that type of distance again was all but a distant memory.

Fast forward to September 2021 and there I was, standing at the start line, preparing to undertake this popular and vibrant running event once again. Looking back, I'd never have imagined I could run this distance ever again; after all, I was almost dead less than 18 months previously! Fulfilling a promise to my donor that I would finish the half-marathon, plus that old memory of missing out on the 2016 event, fuelled me forward and allowed me to push myself and finish at a time of two and a half hours. I was chuffed when I discovered that this was only 45 minutes slower than my previous time of one hour and 45 minutes back when I was fit and healthy!

This makes you realise how amazing the human body really is! My next aim is to complete the 2022 London Marathon, raising money for the British Heart Foundation. The funds raised will go towards funding new advances in treatment for those who are in a similar situation to the one I was in. It has always been an aim of mine to take part in the UK's most iconic marathon, so to do it for the BHF and my donor is an honour.

After that, who knows? Some small triathlons; maybe that goal of completing an Ironman isn't as far out of reach as I first thought?

All I know is that, just as with hardship in life, all it takes is to put one foot in front of the other and keep going.

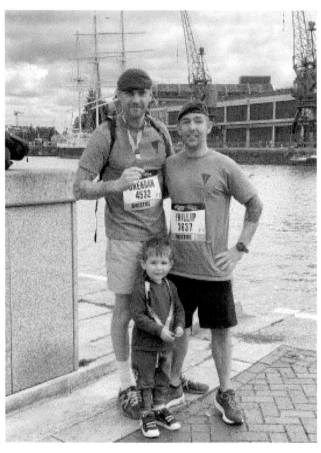

September 2021: Only 18 months after the
heart transplant, I had completed the Bristol
half marathon in two and a half hours.

Resilience

You've heard this word mentioned a lot in my book, so what exactly is resilience? And, more importantly, who am I to tell you about it?

Resilience is defined in the Oxford Learners Dictionaries[3] as: 'The ability of people or things to recover quickly after something unpleasant, such as shock, injury etc. *'He showed great courage and resilience in fighting back from a losing position to win the game.'*

To me, resilience means the ability to cope with change and all the negative feelings that come with it. Resilience is having extra energy ready to deal with change. Some of the foundations for building resilience are diet, exercise and general lifestyle and, later in this chapter, I have included ten things that I aim to use daily to help me feel unstoppable.

Resilience is a word we hear more and more today – and for very good reason. Poor mental health is at its highest level since the coronavirus pandemic started. The mental health charity Mind carried out two surveys of over 10,000 adults aged 25+ and 1,756 young people aged 13-24 and found that 80% and 84% respectively suffered mental distress before or during the pandemic.[4]

The average waiting time for someone in the UK to see

---

3 www.oxfordlearnersdictionaries.com/definition/english/resilience
4https://www.mind.org.uk/media/8962/the-consequences-of-coronavirus-for-mental-health-final-report.pdf

a mental health practitioner is around six months. If you're reading this and feel like you, or someone you know is struggling with their mental health, then please seek professional help. I still struggle with my mental health to this day and will always have periods when it may drop off, or problems may re-occur. I have learnt to use a range of tools to help me manage it, which I will share with you shortly.

For years I bottled up my emotions, until Roxy got me to open up about my past traumas. That was the first step and getting it all off my chest felt like a massive release. Please don't be like me and let your ego make you tell yourself and others that you are 'fine' when, in reality, you are falling apart inside. It takes guts to admit that you have a problem, but it is the first crucial step to healing.

I firmly believe that everyone already has resilience inside themselves. Our ancestors went through many struggles, such as famine, wars and disease. I believe the hardships they endured meant they had resilience in abundance, and likely passed it on to us. Our lives are as comfortable as they have ever been and although we don't have to worry about being hunted, like our ancestors did, we still need tools such as mental toughness and resilience in order to survive and thrive in this modern world. Therefore, with resilience we can resolve our struggles effectively when they arise.

Some people choose to be resilient in order to help them prepare for whatever struggles life has to offer – because we will all face life's challenges at some point in our lives, sometimes when we least expect it. On the other hand, there are people like me who have been forced to be resilient from a young age. Either way, resilience can transform you from a victim mindset and thinking "Why is this happening to me?" to instead thinking "What can I learn from this in order for me to come back stronger?" One of the main differences is that the second person takes a step back, reflects on what they could have done better, accepts the situation for what it is and moves on. I have spent many nights alone, in silence, ruminating over and over until self-realisation took over and I began to replace these negative thoughts with more positive ones.

Resilience is one of the key factors to help you live a better life. As the Buddha once said, "Pain is inevitable, suffering is not." You will grieve lost ones, break ups, getting old etc. Life isn't fair, and unfortunately that's something we all need to learn to accept. Unresolved grief can manifest itself back into your life when you least expect it. In order to heal, it is vital that you process this grief and experience all the unpleasant emotions that go with it.

Here is a very brief overview of the ten tools I try to use every day to help me cope with my past grief and any obstacles that come my way, now and in the future.

1. Journaling. I have to be truthful here. I have only owned a journal since 2018. It is something that I have always seen as a very private affair, so I was scared of having one and leaving it around for someone else to read my deepest, darkest thoughts and judge me. Ridiculous, right?! I'm not sure they would find my barely legitimate writing interesting or even understand it, so they would probably get bored easily and put it down! If you have a partner, be upfront with them about it. You have nothing to hide from those closest to you.

Journaling, even just five to ten minutes in the morning

and evening every day (albeit not on some weekends!), has changed my life. They say happiness comes from within, and all you need is a pen, some paper and the thoughts inside your head. There are no hard and fast rules about what to write; scribble whatever is on your mind.

You will find that getting things down on paper can help you process your thoughts and feelings a lot more clearly. And the more you practise journaling, the more it will become natural to you. Remember that questions are the steering wheel of the mind. If you don't ask the right questions, you won't get the answers you are hoping for. If you find you keep asking yourself the same rubbish questions over and over, change them. For example, "Why did she leave me?" can be changed to "What can I learn from this and how do I make sure I don't make the same mistakes next time?" I find that by asking questions and getting deeper into it, you begin to discover the root cause of why you feel the way that you do – and it may not be why you think it is. You will find that a lot of your worries are not about the actual event itself, but the thoughts that we attach to them.

Other things I write about are how well I sleep, how I want to feel that day, what I want to achieve today that will get me closer to my long-term goals, plus at least three things I am grateful for. My journaling in the evenings is a quick reflection of how the day went, three wins I achieved and planning the next day in advance. This helps me with the next tool.

2. Structured sleep routine. This should come as no surprise, but sleep is essential to feel and function at our best. We spend around a third of our lives sleeping; we can go longer without food than sleep! I know in the past I haven't prioritised sleep and felt that I got away with it because I was young. In Afghanistan we had to adapt to disrupted sleep patterns because of completing watch duties at all hours of the day. The body, you will find, will adapt to a particular sleep routine. It's known as the Circadian rhythm and it helps our bodies to wake up when it's light and feel sleepy when it gets dark. This can be affected by an irregular sleep pattern and too much exposure to screens late at night. For that reason I go to bed at 10pm and rise around 6am, even on weekends. (That's having kids for you…!) I now wear blue filter glasses after 8pm and try to minimise using my phone after that time. Too much of a dopamine high can be achieved from being on social media late at night. That goes for working out late at night, too.

Make sure your bedroom is fairly cool and if you are like me and wake up during the night worrying and overthinking things, prepare the next day's task earlier in the evening, jot down what's worrying you in a notebook and come up with ways to rationalise these sometimes irrational thoughts. I find doing all this helps me to get a good night's sleep.

3. Meditation. People may be shocked to know that I meditate at all, let alone that I do it most days! For me, it is a game changer. If you suffer from anxiety and depression then meditation is proven to reduce this, if done consistently. I am so glad that I started mediation back when I was in hospital and I wish I had discovered it earlier. The biggest things holding me back – and possibly holding you back too – is how it can be perceived by those who are not familiar with it, and not knowing how to do it. I downloaded the Headspace app and bought a year's subscription so I could grasp the basics of breathing – and I practised lots. Some days I didn't feel any benefits and other days my mind moved into a calmer, more positive state. Now I can quite happily meditate on the sofa while Luca is watching a children's programme! Granted, it isn't as good as being in complete silence, so that's why I wake up 15 minutes earlier to get it done first thing. I find it makes me more focused and increases my productivity for the day ahead.

If, like me, you are an overthinker and suffer from anxiety, you have nothing to lose by trying meditation. There are many forms of meditation but I keep it fairly simple, focusing on mindfulness techniques like inhaling through the nose and exhaling through the mouth, switching focus to the rest of the body, saying affirmations in your head in sequence and so on.

If the thought of meditation doesn't appeal to you, then set aside time each day to focus on some deep breathing and I guarantee it will change your state, making you feel better. Ever notice when you are stressed, angry or nervous, your breathing becomes faster and shorter? Focus on slowing down your breathing, which will give you more time to assess the situation. The pay-off may prevent you from acting in a way you might later regret.

4. Exercise. If you want to feel better and live longer, exercise is essential. There are too many benefits to list that we can all gain if we take the time to be more active. Like I said previously, I truly believe that all the years of resistance training and cardiovascular exercise helped my heart to keep me alive as long as it did. If you are sedentary and sit around all day, your body will tighten up and your posture will suffer. This can lead to lower back pain over time, with tight hip flexors being the main culprit. Same as spending hours a day looking down at a phone screen will give you neck pains. To keep these little niggles at bay, you need to carry out some exercise and mobility or stretches regularly, preferably daily! It has to be something sustainable that you enjoy.

For me, my love of exercise began with playing football as a six-year-old. Back then, I didn't consider it a form of exercise and I still don't. With exercise there are no quick results; progress takes a long time but it is all worth it. There is information on exercise in some of the earlier chapters, but always remember that everyone has different genes and factors affecting how fast they progress, so don't compare your results to anyone else's, or compare yourself against others about anything, full stop!

5. Diet – both physical and mental. Two diets, you say?! One is bad enough! The physical side is that you are what you eat. From how you look, your weight, hair, skin and nails to how you feel, food plays a huge role. If you eat a lot of processed foods and refined sugar then you will feel like crap! On top of that, the higher risks of coronary heart disease, stroke and type 2 diabetes are all associated with being overweight and eating too much saturated fat, salt and sugary processed foods.

On the other hand, if you eat a balanced diet, including minimally processed foods, along with fruits and vegetables, with plenty of water, I guarantee you will feel and look better. You are what you eat is true for a reason!

By mental diet, I mean assessing what input you are exposed to on a daily basis. Do you check social media or the news as soon as you wake up? If so, that could put you in a negative mood before the day's even begun! If you associate with friends who are negative and gossip about others, chances are it will rub off on you. Have you spoken to a happy positive person and immediately felt better by the good vibes they give off? Then you need to spend more time around these types of people. Same with the programmes you watch on TV. Watching reality shows where the aim is essentially to treat each other badly in order to win money and boost ratings seems morally wrong to me. Take a good look at the environment you are in. Like I said earlier, my life was heading towards mediocrity, spearheaded by heavy drink and drug use, until I made the decision to distance myself from it all and join the army.

6. Read personal development books. It wasn't until about the age of 25 that I started reading regularly. I was in a Waterstones in London while I was providing security for the 2012 Olympic Games when I spotted out of my eye a book called The Chimp Paradox by Dr Steve Peters. I am not sure why I was so drawn to it, but I am a firm believer that the universe is sending you signals each day, and it's up to you to find them. My love of reading personal development books started there, and not long afterwards, I bought my first Kindle. This travels with me everywhere!

There is a huge amount of information in books that can help improve any area of your life. I have read that the average CEO reads around 52 books a year. That's one a week! And if a CEO can find time in their busy schedule to read a book a week then we can too. I tend to read before going to bed as I find it is a great way to unwind. If reading is not your thing, why not try an Audible version of a book instead, or listen to inspiring podcasts, which are also free!

If the thought of reading about personal development doesn't excite you, how about a book on a subject you want to learn about, or a subject that could benefit your career prospects? Now and again I find myself studying a subject that may or may not benefit me financially but is more for interest and to broaden my knowledge. When I visited Italy with my oldest son Reggie, I think we both fell in love with the place, the culture and the food. This led to me learning more about the Romans, which then led me to discover the great Stoic philosophers, such as Marcus Aurelius, Seneca and Epictetus. Much of their philosophy is still prevalent to this very day; Marcus Aurelius' writing on meditations is one such book that can change your perspective and how you see life and the events happening around you.

7. Limiting social media. Social media can be a great tool for keeping in touch with family and friends, searching for information and sharing positive memories. However, there are many negative sides to using too much social media. This can include comparison with others, leading to envy, jealousy and depression.

If you are relying on external validation by posting something online to receive likes, you will be disappointed internally when you don't get as many as you hoped for. Being online means less face to face contact, which can result in social anxiety or cyber bullying – and don't forget how distracting it can be. How many times have you thought you would check it for ten minutes and next thing you know, it is late into the evening! I think we have all done this at one point or another because social media is addictive. Every time you scroll down you get lots of little dopamine hits and eventually it wears you out. This in turn affects our sleep and the quality of it.

I feel that a lot of the time we are checking our phones on autopilot, constantly looking for messages or updates. Social media apps are designed to keep you purposely scrolling for as long as possible. I have an app blocker app that I use for certain times of the day and I turn off notifications on my phone so I am not distracted when I am trying to focus on spending time with my boys or working. I have found that reducing my time online, especially within the first hour of waking up, has significantly reduced my stress

8. Morning and evening routines. This is key and really helps me make the most of each day. I wake up slightly earlier than I need to. Don't worry, you don't necessarily have to! The reason I do it is because I can enjoy an hour first thing to myself with no distractions. That means no checking my phone and no TV in that first hour! It is designed to prime you for the day ahead and to prepare you to handle any setbacks that are out of your control throughout the day. For example, if I get stuck in traffic on the way to work, I am usually much calmer if I have carried out my morning routine that day.

My routine usually consists of meditation for 10-15 minutes, two glasses of water, some light mobility and stretching, followed by my journal and some reading, if I have time before Luca wakes up. In the evening, I do some studying or reading and generally settle down in order to prime myself for sleep. That could mean reducing phone time, having a shower and then finishing with my journal to reflect on how the day went and have my next day planned out ready to go. However, my routine is not set in stone as some days I may be unwell or Luca may wake up early.

Your routines will be unique to you, but it should be easy and it should put you in a calm state, ready to tackle the day ahead. If you are checking the news or social media first thing in the morning, then you are potentially exposing yourself to negativity from the start of the day.

The main aim here is to turn it into a habit and not focus on perfection. Just doing one or two things on your morning or evening routine can have a big impact in the long term.

9. Writing down goals. We all have goals in life, whether it is to be a great parent, become a homeowner, lose weight etc. But many of us lose sight of these goals because we don't write them down! I remember my goal was once to be a homeowner by the age of 30. I didn't achieve that goal. Do I let it define my success? No. It is drilled into British society that we should achieve certain landmarks by a certain age. Marriage by this age and children by that age. But everyone's metrics are different. My circumstances made a big difference but ultimately I didn't do what was required to be in a position to buy a house. I just expected to somehow muster up a decent sized deposit by age 30; I didn't factor in anything else about the process of owning a home. It wasn't my highest value, just a 'be nice to' dream.

Being a great dad and making sure my boys don't experience the same upbringing I had is my highest value. They are reliant on me and look to me for guidance, meaning that my role as a father needs to consist of investing my time and energy into making sure they have a great start in life. Making sure I don't turn to alcohol like my parents did; making their environment a warm and loving place where they feel safe and can prosper. Notice that the original sentence referred to them not experiencing the same upbringing as me. That is my metric for success. For others, it may be making sure their child goes to university and becomes a doctor. Of course, that would be a 'nice to' dream, but for me it is something my boys can decide for themselves, once I've helped put the appropriate foundations in place for them to follow their own ideas of success.

One of the most common ways of setting goals is the SMART method. I have written and rewritten my goals hundreds of times over the years, changing them as I evolve and learning from past mistakes, which is most likely a lack of planning on my part. Once you have a longer-term goal, you can reverse engineer the steps required to achieve that goal so they can be used as checkpoints, if you like. An example of a SMART goal in its most basic form would be this:

- ✓ **Specific:** Lose 10lbs
- ✓ **Measurable:** Using scales at home, I will take daily measurements and use a seven-day average to get a better reflection, as opposed to weighing myself once a week (as weight on the scales can fluctuate wildly depending on many factors including hydration levels, sleep, hormones etc).
- ✓ **Achievable:** I was 10lbs lighter before so I know this is achievable. (I went from 84kg at the start of my hospital stay and came out at 59kg!)
- ✓ **Realistic:** Here it is useful to use something like the SWOT analysis.
  - **Strengths** – I have previous knowledge and experience in losing weight.

- **Weaknesses** – Not sticking to eating well, emotional eating, falling ill and ending up in hospital again.
- **Opportunities** – When the boys are away, it means I have time to work out, either at my local gym or using the gym equipment I have at home.
- **Threats** – I currently have Luca every morning and evening, so it will not be possible to leave him and go to the gym. A contingency plan is having some weights at home, which I have in the living room, so I can still do weights in the evenings.
- **Time-Based:** Six months, or a specific date. Setting a deadline is incredibly important as you're not going to create any urgency if there's no end date! Referring back to the reverse engineering part, this also allows you to put steps in place. So, if my goal was to lose 10lbs in six months, my halfway goal would be 5lbs in three months and so on, down to weekly and daily goals bringing me closer to the end goal.

This brings us to discovering your 'why': something that is true to your values and not what someone else expects of you. Take some time to discover what it is that makes you excited to get out of bed in the mornings. That will keep you going when motivation runs out.

This also ties in with your life mission. This acts as your North Star and guides you towards what you really want out of life. It assesses whether the daily decisions and habits in life are pushing you towards your North Star or taking you further away. Find your North Star!

10. Learning to love yourself. This is something I have struggled with pretty much my whole life. Poor mental health has a way of giving you low self-worth and somehow, a feeling that you are not as worthy as everyone else. Everyone is equal and unique in their own special way. Remember that you have no idea what someone else is going through, so it's best just to be kind. Controlling your emotions, especially empathy, can help you see things from another person's point of view. I have heard the saying many times to 'put your own oxygen mask on when on a flight before helping others', and it's true; you have to put yourself first.

At first you might think that sounds selfish; it almost goes against our intuition to serve and help others first. But how can you help other people if you are not helping yourself? If I want my boys to have the best version of me that lives around the longest then I have to put myself first. You can't serve from an empty cup – so make sure your cup is full first!

Of course, there may be some exceptions to this. For example, if I only had enough food to feed either me or my boys, then of course I would feed them and go hungry myself.

The bottom line that I'm trying to get at is that I'm willing to put the hard work in so it doesn't have to come to that. Your internal dialogue is so important and what you tell yourself, your mind will believe. If you are constantly speaking negatively to yourself all the time, learn to love yourself, be proud of who you are when you look in the mirror, prioritise self-care and don't be afraid to treat yourself from time to time. You are worth it!

You may already do some of these habits yourself. And if you do, then you will know the benefits they provide! It may sound exhausting to do all of these every day on top of looking after children and working full time, but this is where effective planning comes into place. If you are low on energy some days, the aim is to forget about perfectionism and just do something. Even if you only do a couple of the activities on the list, it is still taking you a step closer to your goals and is better than nothing.

This is just my personal list, of course. You can amend the activities or swap them for something that provides similar benefits. For example, if personal development books are not your thing, replace it with something that benefits you and provides a chance for improvement, such as something that works your brain like a puzzle or some research on the internet about a subject you are interested in. There are so many online courses you can do from your phone that won't break the bank. I'm currently learning Italian because I fell in love with the place when I visited and it is another challenge to test myself on.

The main thing is consistency, and if you don't like your routine then chances are you won't stick with it in the long run. Habits are formed when we make them easy to do. They say it takes 21 days to form a habit. I believe it can take more or less time depending on the individual and/or the habit in question. There will be times when you are unwell and you won't want to do anything but lie on the sofa – and there's nothing wrong with that. I have to have a day off each week in order to recharge. But you must make sure that any bad habits don't creep back in again. Say you fall off track and eat more than your body needs; instead of packing it all in thinking that your healthy eating plan has gone out of the window, get back on track quickly in order to break that cycle and help build resilience in the process.

If I had to pick out the three main habits that will help you overcome most things in life, they would undoubtedly be sleep, eating well and exercising. All three are vital for feeling and performing at your best, and then you can build other habits on top of those.

Organ Donation

For me, along with all the other transplant survivors past and present, their donors and their families, this chapter is something that needs to be written. Quite simply, this book wouldn't have existed without my donor. Without my donated heart, I wouldn't be alive to write this now and my family wouldn't have the extra time they have had with me up to now. It is one of the many reasons I am extremely grateful every day.

The NHS states that one organ donor can save up to nine lives through multiple organ and tissue donation[5]. You may have noticed that since 2020, the UK has adopted an 'opt out' system, also known as Max and Keira's Law, in honour of a boy who received a heart transplant from the girl who donated it. This law means that everyone who passes away could potentially become an organ donor unless they have chosen to opt out.

I know there has been some criticism about this, and I have seen some online comments along the lines of "I don't want my body being used like that after my death" and "It's another form of control by the government".

Of course, everyone is entitled to their own opinion, but you never know when you or a family member may need an organ transplant. The ultimate decision still lies with the family after a death.

---

5 https://www.save9lives.com/nhs-facts

There is currently a big shortage of organ donors in the UK and the waiting lists for kidney, liver and heart transplants are longer than ever before. The survival rate of a heart transplant recipient has risen a lot in the years since the very first heart transplant way back in 1967.

"On December 3, 1967, 53-year-old Louis Washkansky received the first human heart transplant at Groote Schuur Hospital in Cape Town, South Africa.

Washkansky, a South African grocer dying from chronic heart disease, received the transplant from Denise Darvall, a 25-year-old woman who was fatally injured in a car accident. Surgeon Christiaan Barnard, who trained at the University of Cape Town and in the United States, performed the revolutionary medical operation. The technique Barnard employed was initially developed by a group of American researchers in the 1950s. American surgeon Norman Shumway achieved the first successful heart transplant, in a dog, at Stanford University in California in 1958.

After Washkansky's surgery, he was given drugs to suppress his immune system and keep his body from rejecting the heart. These drugs also left him susceptible to sickness, however, and he died 18 days later from double pneumonia. Despite the setback, Washkansky's new heart had functioned normally until his death.[6]"

Due to technological advances in science and equipment, along with better knowledge of how to treat transplant patients with medication etc., some heart

---

6 First human heart transplant. Author: History.com Editors, original publication date July 21, 2010. https://www.history.com/this-day-in-history/first-human-heart-transplant

transplant patients are living an extra 35+ years. Simply amazing! And then there are the BiVADs and ECMO machines, which definitely saved my life and kept me alive long enough to receive a new heart.

As of 1st April 2022, there were 6,269 people on the organ waiting list in the UK and 3,401 people have received an organ transplant since April 2021[7]. By agreeing to becoming an organ donor, you are helping to save the lives of ordinary people like myself. The hospital will still do all they can to save your life if you are in hospital, and you will be treated with dignity and respect throughout the process.

There are also strict criteria in place to deal with dying patients and organs are not removed until these criteria are met. Of course, you don't have to be deceased to be an organ donor. For example, you can still donate a kidney and survive with just one. Transplant laws in the UK state that organs are a precious gift passed on to those most in need, and this law also bans the sale of organs and tissue.

In the UK you can register to become an organ donor; you may even have seen those pink cards that let others know you are registered. It is essential that you let your family members know of your decision. For more information about the NHS Organ Donation and Transplantation Register, please go to https://www.organdonation.nhs.uk/register-to-donate/

Don't forget, you can opt out at any time, or even get somebody else to make a decision on your behalf. Ultimately, it will be your family or next of kin that make

---

7.https://www.organdonation.nhs.uk/helping-you-to-decide/about-organ-donation/statistics-about-organ-donation/

the final decision. I know it is an extremely difficult conversation to have with your family, but it is best to leave them certain of your wishes.

My hope is that by writing this book, I can convince just one person to decide to donate their organs after death. I know it was my donor's dying wish and I want to honour his decision by being the best father I can be and give something back to the world.

Conclusion

I procrastinated a lot writing this book. I wrote it, then rewrote it. Memories were often too painful to revisit. However, this was all totally necessary in order to manage the years of grief that I had stored up in my head. This unprocessed grief had a hold over my life and would often rear its ugly head at random times. Now I have the tools and experience to deal with these recurring negative thought patterns, I feel my grief is a passenger and is staying with me for the ride. Thinking about my transplant journey, and even going back to the smallest details from my childhood, can invoke scary feelings of that near-fateful time in hospital. I also dwelled on my downward spiral from being a fit and athletic commando to barely being able to leave the house. I kept telling myself I'd start writing next week, or have some other fear-induced thought like "What if I'm not capable of writing a book?" or "What if nobody buys it?" The answer, I told myself, was that there is no perfect time to get started; action was, in fact, the only answer I needed. If it fails, at least I have tried my best with the skills I have at this moment in time.

All we can do is banish that fear of failure that's holding us back and try and improve as we go along. Certain failure would have been not trying at all, so at least I have tried – and if I fail, I'll still be happier because of the process that came through writing this book. And if you have read this far, it must be ok!

The setbacks I have faced in my life and the lessons I have learnt up to now have helped build my resilience. Throughout my journey, it would have been very easy to play the victim card and say that I can't do this or that, but I don't think that is inside me. That is why I push myself each day to be the best version of myself – so my family gets the best version of me as well. I've had good days and bad days up to this point; emotions change daily, such as motivation, which comes and goes. Therefore it's best to accept that there will be some days when you are not feeling your best and practise self-care rather than beating yourself up about it.

Anything worthwhile in life takes time and today we are in so much of a rush, looking for the quick fix and trying to find the shortcut – but we often find ourselves ending up back at square one. While in hospital, I read several books on my Kindle about personal development, and also listened to many podcasts that I wish I had discovered many years ago. The information contained in them helped me grow exponentially as a person. Some of the daily habits I have included in this book I was already doing naturally, and others have been discovered through reading or listening to the wealth of information available out there. Chances are you may already be doing them yourself.

Remember that success varies from person to person. All too often we affiliate success with having lots of money, a nice house and a flash car. That is not always the case. Find out what is important to you rather than what you think others expect of you. One of the most rewarding things we can do in life is to give something back to others. Whatever situation you find yourself in, there is already somebody worse off than you. When I was extremely ill and spent so long in hospital, I had no income to make the payments for our house and bills. It's thanks to my local community and our friends and their generosity that we had a home to go back to.

After my transplant I organised a fundraising football match. It was a great feeling to give something back to others and be able to raise over £1,000 for Royal Papworth Hospital. And it was a dream come true to be able to play alongside my oldest boy, Reggie. This was something that seemed impossible way back in the despair of 2019 and early 2020.

The mind is the most powerful tool we possess and it is our responsibility to harness it to its true potential. Resilience is in all of us and I hope that by reading this book and working on yourself daily, you will have the skills available to tackle whatever life throws at you, now and in the future. You are stronger than you realise and can recover from almost any setback and prosper again. Please don't make the same mistake I made and not live a life that is true to your values. Don't wait for a life-changing event like I went through before you make your physical and mental health your highest priority. Make sure you are the best you can be for yourself and all those around you.

I feel it is best to end this book on a positive note. After all the setbacks I've had in life, I've learnt that organ donation is one of the most selfless and wonderful things you can do. I am one of the very lucky ones to receive a new heart and every organ donor should receive the utmost respect for passing on the gift of life in order for those like me to have this second chance.

By the way, now I do believe in miracles.

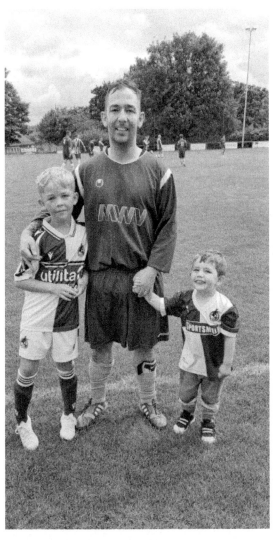

August 2021: A dream come true being able to play football again, especially with my oldest son Reggie, and raising over £1000 in the process for the Royal Papworth Hospital Charity.

Acknowledgements

Thank you to my family, especially my boys, Reggie and Luca, who have been so brave and for being my inspiration to push myself every day as well as keeping me on my toes!

Thank you to Roxanne for being there at the time. Without you, I wouldn't have made it to receive my heart.

Thank you to Sheila and Gill for looking after Luca throughout his life, especially while we were in hospital.

Thank you to all my friends and the community of Yate and beyond for their support to my family and me when I was ill and afterwards as well.

Thank you to the staff at the Royal Papworth Hospital, who saved my life on numerous occasions, as well as the Bristol Royal Infirmary staff for the treatment I received before being admitted to Papworth.

Thank you to 29 Commando Regiment for their continued support during my hospital stay and beyond, not to mention for building up my resilience over the years!

Thank you to the military charity SSAFA and The Royal Artillery Trust Fund for their donations to help my family and me during difficult times.

Thank you to my beta readers: Alex Willer, Bradley Hackett, Nicola Henderson, Steven Woodruff, Michael Pash and Thomas Davies.

Thank you to The Proof Fairy, Alison Thompson, for working her magic with the editing, proofreading, formatting and cover design for this book; she's someone I would definitely recommend to help you turn your book dreams into reality!

Last but not least, I want to thank my organ donor for making that selfless decision to sign up for organ donation, along with their family for making the final decision for their child/family member to donate their organs. If it wasn't for them, I wouldn't be here today and this book wouldn't have been possible. I am forever in your debt and grateful each day for the precious gift I have received. I love you all and God bless.

About the Author

I grew up in a small town called Yate, which is just north of the city of Bristol, where I still reside now with my two boys Reggie and Luca, and dog Pedro. After a difficult upbringing, when I was 14 my mum died from a rare form of heart disease, unbeknownst to me until 15 years later. My mum's death left me an anxious and depressed teenager. I joined the army at 18 and went on to serve 12 years as a gunner in 29 Commando Regiment Royal Artillery. I served in two tours of Afghanistan and various exercises around the world, including Norway, the Falkland Islands and the US. My hobbies include running, weightlifting, reading and watching football. My aim is to make the most of my second chance at life. This includes being the best dad that I can be, promoting organ donation and raising money for charity by taking part in physical challenges.

Printed in Great Britain
by Amazon

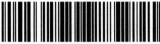

80526721R00098